# The Midlife Bible

## A Woman's Survival Guide

by
Michael Goodman, M.D.

Robert D. Reed Publishers • San Francisco, CA

**Robert D. Reed Publishers**
P.O. 1992, 1380 Face Rock Drive
Bandon, OR 97411
Phone: 650-994-6570 • Fax: -6579
E-mail: 4bobreed@msn.com
web site: www.rdrpublishers.com


Typesetter: **Barbara Kruger**
Cover Designer: **Julia Gaskill**


ISBN 1-931741-32-8

Library of Congress Control Number 2003091191


Manufactured, typeset and printed in the United States of America

# Dedication

"For my Family and my Patients"

# Acknowledgments

"The Midlife Bible arose from seeds sewn by my realization of the failure of the managed care system and its health care providers to adequately deal with the difficulties midlife imposes on many women. These seeds were watered by the enlightenment and education generated by the participants in the 2001 and 2002 annual meetings of the North American Menopause Society and nourished by the countless brave souls who have written articles, books and researched alternatives for good health care for midlife women.

Without the steadfast transcription, online skills and general good humor of Beverly Sykes, this book would never have seen the light of day. Without the interest of Ann Louise Gittleman, PhD., I would not have found a publisher. Without the steadfast work and direction of my publicists, Danek Kaus and Maryglenn McCombs, no one would know about this book.

I thank my friend and collegue William Parker, M.D., as well as Elizabeth Lee Vliet, M.D., and Maida Taylor, M.D., whose thoughtful reading of "The Bible" and constructive comments have made this a better book. I thank Nancy Alspaugh and Marilyn Kentz (those fearless women!) for their insight and philosophy. The clever cartoons of Dee Adams take this book from "the drab" to "the droll."

I thank Nyna Nelson, F.N.P., for her knowledge of compounding, a bit of which has hopefully rubbed off onto me.

Most of all, I am indebted to the patients who braved the domain of "Independent Practice" in our health care-managed world and provided the impetus and ideas for this book. I love you all. I hope I have taught as much as I have learned.

# Contents

# Foreword

"Midlife" women's health isn't a simple subject. This is a time when change impacts all dimensions of our lives. But at the most fundamental biological level, it is a time when our unique hormone changes are creating incredible and complex interactions between the physical, psychological, social and spiritual aspects of our being. As a physician specializing in women's health for the last twenty years, and focusing my work on the nuances and complexities of the multitudinous ways that our ovarian hormones are linked to the function of every cell and tissue of our brain and body, I have personally treated thousands of women looking for ways to restore optimal health and hormone balance. I have conducted research, written books, and have taught seminars for health professionals and consumers around the county on these overlooked hormone connections in women's health and how crucial it is for those of us in medicine to take these issues seriously.

Yet, I write this foreword not just as a physician and scientist. I also write as a woman who has been there with the tribulations and challenges of "menopause." I am a "midlife woman" who is on the journey, along with you readers. I have lived it firsthand. I know what it is like to go through the tumult of erratic cycles and feel like my body belongs to an alien creature. I know what it is like to feel "sharp" and then suddenly feel like a switch has been flipped and my brain turned to mush, trapping and holding my words and thoughts hostage with yet another hormone shift. I have also been "a patient," needing several surgeries that added to the health challenges and gave me more "learning experiences." I know what it is like to struggle to find hormone balance amidst life stresses, a changing body and multiple medical problems. It isn't a simple matter. There isn't one simple answer that works for every woman. What works for you will be different from what works for your friend. Women facing the challenges of midlife have much to consider. It IS a life-changing time—positive, negative, and all points in-between these opposites.

The problem is that women's health care has been fragmented over many separate specialties, with each specialist treating a set of symptoms belonging to a different body part. Women see multiple physicians and get multiple medications, but rarely do physicians take into account—or check-baseline measures of our ovarian hormones, or the profound connections between ovarian hormone and other body symptoms we have, and how we cope with day-to-day stresses. Women *know* there is a connection, yet their insights and observations are dismissed and discounted. The end result is that many women feel devalued and disconnected from their physicians at the very time in our lives when we most need a knowledgeable, concerned, compassionate physician *partner* in our health journey.

Dr. Goodman's book, *The Midlife Bible: A Woman's Survival Guide,* helps provide a guide to the many different options out there today— hormonal, other types of prescription medications, herbal remedies, over-the-counter supplements, and dietary and lifestyle approaches. From his career as a gynecologist helping women over many years, Dr. Goodman has compiled an overview of the variety of options he has found effective. The goal of *The Midlife Bible* is not to give a definitive answer or "how-to" guide, but rather to give woman a broad picture of the many approaches available today to help us maintain, and improve, our health and well-being. No book can tell every woman what to do, and no one approach will be right for every woman. Dr. Goodman describes many different paths, so that a woman can choose approaches suitable for her needs. Some women will want to consider using hormones, others won't. Some will need antidepressants, and others won't. Some women will do fine with herbal products, others won't. The key here, as Dr. Goodman so clearly points out, is for each woman to become educated about the options, take an inventory of her needs and preferences, have a thorough and objective evaluation of risks and health goals, and become empowered to make choices right for *her.*

Today, with many options to help you feel better, women deserve better answers than they have typically received in our fragmented, time-pressured health care system today. For those who want more detailed information on various subjects, Dr. Goodman has provided a list of resources that you should find helpful, and I have also described many of these issues and options in my own books.

Hormones—and their connections in how we think and feel and function—have been my life's work in medicine. The summer of 2002—and months since—brought a maelstrom of negative, frightening headlines about "hormones" and "hormone replacement therapy" (HRT). The headlines screamed that "hormones" or "estrogen" increases the risk of breast cancer, heart disease and dementia. But they *don't* tell you that such headlines are based on only one study, using Prempro®, the *combination* of estrogens from pregnant mares' urine (Premarin®) and synthetic progestin (Provera®) given to elderly women with multiple medical problems: 66% were significantly overweight, 36% had high blood pressure, and 16% had a family member with breast cancer!

Neither Premarin® nor Provera® provide hormones identical to what our bodies make naturally, a point rarely mentioned in the coverage. Why do risks found with one non-human hormone product get applied to *all* hormone preparations, even though they are chemically different?. We don't see that happening in any other field of medicine, or with any other class of medications. Why does it happen with women's hormones? We don't see such sensationalized, frightening headlines about men's testosterone. All this furor and alarmist headlines have made women of all ages terrified of "hormones"—even young women are afraid to take birth control pills. Yet there are many well-studied, alternative, bioidentical (or "natural") forms of hormones available, with fewer negative effects. What is really going on here? How do you make sense of the bewildering maze of information and conflicting reports as you navigate this journey? As you read through Dr. Goodman's guide to midlife, keep in mind some important facts that often get overlooked in most healthcare settings:

1. Physicians rarely measure hormone levels when women are in their prime and feel well to have a baseline for later comparison. And doctors typically don't measure women's hormone levels to see whether medications are achieving the desired result. Doctors just say "they vary" and don't bother to see *how* levels vary with symptoms and various body changes. Yet, insidious decline in ovarian hormone production wreaks havoc throughout our bodies, in every organ system, including the brain. It is not clear to me why many doctors don't think checks of ovarian hormone levels are necessary. The same physicians would not dream of starting thyroid, or diabetes or cholesterol medications without having baseline laboratory measures of TSH, glucose, or lipids. Part of the problem is due to doctors' *assumptions* that "vague" symptoms such as insomnia, anxiety, low libido, and depressed mood occur because of psychological reactions to the "stresses" of midlife, feelings of lost femininity, or fear of aging. This focus on assumed psychological issues completely overlooks the physical hormone effects on brain chemistry and function. Loss of ovarian hormones that play crucial metabolic roles throughout our body—from sex to weight to energy level to memory and mood and sleep and pain regulation—can be very disturbing. When women and their doctors don't have this information, they are often given treatment recommendations that are ineffective. Women need to be their own advocates, and need to learn what to ask for in the way of tests. This book helps you do that.

2. Even if women *do* decide to start hormone therapy, most still do not get "optimal" replacement of their ovarian hormones. The usual approach is to simply give estrogen, usually Premarin®, which provides very little of the 17-beta estradiol our bodies have always made, and need. Testosterone is rarely replaced. Testosterone enhances energy level, libido, sense of well-being and mood, bone and muscle formation and also (along with estradiol) improves the vaginal tissue to relieve dryness that causes pain during sex. The vast majority of women who may benefit *still* are not offered

testosterone therapy. And there is typically no individualization of type, route or dose of hormones suggested. It doesn't have to be this way. Most women are amazed at the degree of well-being that can return with the right type of hormone replacement, the right delivery approach and optimal levels, along with an integrated approach to diet, exercise, and stress management. But if no one is checking your hormone levels with reliable blood tests, the hormone cause of symptoms is missed. Fatigue, headaches, depression, insomnia, loss of sex drive, and other symptoms are then more likely labeled depression, chronic fatigue, anxiety or stress.

3. The hormone furor of the past few years has unnecessarily frightened many women into being afraid of taking "hormones." Yet what is overlooked is that the product being discussed in the headlines is *not* our natural estrogen or natural progesterone. It is a mixture of horse-derived estrogens and a potent synthetic progestin that can have many negative effects. In the Women's Health Initiative (WHI) study, the estrogen-only group (women who had previously had hysterectomy) was *not* stopped because this group was not showing the negative outcomes found in the combined estrogen-progestin (Prempro®) group. The media seemed to ignore this crucial point. There is *good* news about the emerging research showing many benefits of estradiol—and testosterone—with cyclic progesterone for women who have a uterus, for many dimensions of women's well-being and health. Sadly, such positive findings often don't get reported in the media that seems to focus on sensationalizing the negative and promoting fear.

I know there is a better way to prevent such disastrous outcomes that rob women of their sexuality, their sense of womanhood, and their body-mind-spirit health. If you have spent years suffering, not feeling well, and going from doctor to doctor trying to find a way to relieve symptoms and to feel better, start your journey to regaining your well-being by having your hormone levels properly checked. Then read and become informed about the many prescription options, lifestyle choices, and complementary approaches to help you regain hormone balance and health. There is hope, and help available. You deserve to have your health concerns taken seriously. Become your own advocate. Take charge of this journey. Make midlife the great time of life. It is your gateway to the second half of adult life we are privileged to be able to live—make it healthy, happy, productive and full of zest!

Elizabeth Lee Vliet, M.D., Author of
*It's My OVARIES, Stupid!* (Scribner, 2003)
*Screaming to Be Heard: Hormone Connections Women Suspect and Doctors Still Ignore* (M. Evans, 1995, Revised edition 2001)
Women, Weight and Hormones (M.Evans, 2001)

# Preface

Short and sweet.

I enjoyed the heck out of writing this book. My goal was to put down in easily readable and not too long-winded form all the information necessary for a woman and her partner to inform themselves of the options available to ease her passage through menopause.

What I've learned and what my patients have taught me in 33 years of medical practice (the last 10 of which have been directed toward peri-menopausal/menopausal issues) are the stuff that make up these pages. Peri-menopause; premenstrual syndrome; hormone replacement therapy and alternatives; health enhancement; the spectre of breast cancer; bone density; sexuality issues; bleeding problems; stress and fatigue states; pelvic floor problems; how to get what you need from the health care system; what's on the horizon. It's all here.

No axes to grind. No "my way or the highway." Just an honest appraisal of all the methods out there and where they may fit into your equation, and a very complete resource section (both on-line and books) to guide those seeking more in-depth and reflective information in each specific area.

Informed decision making for better health care!

Enjoy!

*If you educate a man, you educate a person. And if you educate a woman, you educate a family.*
—Rudy Manikan
(Indian Church Leader)

*Life is Nothing until it is lived; but it is yours to make sense of, and the value of it is nothing other than the sense you choose.*
—Jean Paul Sartre,
*Existentialism & Humanism*

# INTRODUCTION

## "Why this Book?"

A few years ago, after I gave up on private practice (after 25 years), in part because of the restrictions on patient care self-imposed on the medical profession in their love/hate relationship with HMOs, I began doing part time work in the U.S.'s largest HMO, "Kaiser" (Permanente Medical Group). Kaiser was "backed up" for routine gyn appointments for over six months and was willing to part with some cash (just a little!) to find someone who would help with that backload by doing annual exams and helping with "routine" gyn patients.

Since my other "job" at that time was as an obstetrical hospital intensivist with a group of perinatalogists (the specialty that focuses on the period around the time of birth) which provided me 24 hours of a non-stop obstetrical rollercoaster (with side-dishes of gyn disasters), I thought this low-key office work would provide a suitable counterpoint.

I was greatly enjoying my self-structured, post-private practice routine of *locum tenens* (working as a substitute) and in-hospital ob intensivist work. The realm of independent private practice in the brave new (HMO) world was a memory. I would never enter that arena again.

Well, the lion's share of my work at Kaiser involved annual exams and midlife problems in a group of people deemed as problematic in the world of managed care (they took too much TIME): women in their 40s and 50s.

Now, although I respect Kaiser for so successfully and stably providing quality, low cost medical care for so many years, where they (and the entire managed care system) slip is the provision of care to/for women at midlife and other individual situations which require time, patience, and the ability of the practitioner to listen <u>to</u> and talk <u>with</u> (not at) a client to allow participation in an individually crafted therapeutic regimen.

It is virtually impossible in the managed care world of 15-minute office visits for a patient to participate in a therapeutic regimen crafted by an individual well versed in the alternative regimens for the several travails that midlife provides.

"Routine stuff," colds, cuts and bruises, annual health maintenance exams, vaginitis checks, high blood pressure, minor infections, etc., etc.— anything which can be handled in a minimal-exchange 10-15 minute visit is well treated by managed care (which in my area accounts for 80-90% of medical care). But within the system there simply is not enough time or interest (and frequently not the knowledge) necessary to properly work with women undergoing midlife passage and to craft a preventative and therapeutic package to work for the individual (and make it malleable enough to change with the passage of time).

I left this assignment with Kaiser-Permanente at their Antioch, California, facility after six months. When, however, I asked for a letter of reference for a position at another Kaiser facility, my "chief" demurred, stating that I "took too much time with my patients," and "did too much ultrasound." The worst part, however, according to her, was that after I left, the patients I had seen were not happy with their subsequent providers. It seemed I had taken more time with them, listened to them, actually answered their questions, and allowed them to participate in a therapeutic plan; altogether NOT in the managed care treatment mode. In short, I had not become "Kaiserized" (..."managed care-ized").

In this context, I realized that health care for women, providing the time and surroundings to help, enable, and empower this passage, was simply <u>not available</u> in the two-million plus geographic area in which I lived.

It was at this point that the need for a "listening" practice, with easy availability of prolonged office visits, first came to mind. Out of this realization, "Caring for Women" was born and I re-entered, as an independent practitioner, the arena of private practice.

In this context, I began perusing the presently available literature relating to the experience of feminine midlife. I found:

1.  Excellent, thorough books on peri-menopause (the months or years prior to menopause)
2.  Excellent, thorough books on menopause.
3.  Excellent, thorough books on natural/naturopathic/nutritional/herbal therapies.
4.  Excellent, thorough books on PMS

Many of these books are well written ±300 page affairs and are excellent references for women desiring to know more on these specific areas.

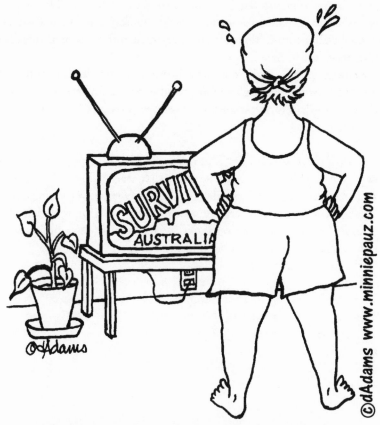

**HA! What's a few bugs and sleeping on the ground? Let them try 5+years of hot flashes, insomnia and crawly skin! That's a REAL challenge!**

Nowhere, however, in the over 50 texts I reviewed, did I see a complete but concise, informative, readable, up to date, inexpensive book that covered <u>ALL</u> of the issues of feminine midlife. PMS. Peri-menopause and menopause. "Natural," nutritional, lifestyle and hormonal approaches. Bone density problems. Sexuality issues. Fatigue states. Stress. Vulvar pain problems. Incontinence and prolapse (when the uterus falls from its normal position). Late childbearing. Relationship issues. What's brand new and what's on the horizon. How, as a midlife woman, to get what you need from the managed care system. One that specifically helped the reader to see the path that was safest and best for her.

This is <u>not</u> just another book on menopause. *The Midlife Bible* is an immediately up-to-date cover of most all of the issues to be encountered by a woman passing through midlife. It is an excellent educational overview. A place to start. It's all here.

This is also a book that is very much for, and can (and should) be read by the midlife woman's partner as well, and which, I am confident, will go a long way towards informing and reconnecting men and women with their midlife partners.

"THE DOCTOR IS IN!" This is a story where <u>everyone</u> wins. Midlife is not rocket science. It is a natural, normal passage that we all, women and men alike, go through. (Admittedly, this book is written with female midlife in mind. However, it is every bit as much for men as for their female partners.) There are so many options available! An understanding of these alternatives, along with additional understanding of "what the heck is going on" is the purpose of this book.

*Like a bird on a wire, like a drunk in a midnight choir*
*I have tried, in my way, to be free*
                    —Leonard Cohen,
                    in *Bird on a Wire*

# CHAPTER ONE

## THE FLOW THROUGH MIDLIFE
"Riding the Wave"

The passage through midlife for a woman is, I think, rather like surfing. A lot of paddling, sometimes sun, sometimes clouds. Always salt water. Waiting, treading water. Then riding the wave. Hopefully cruising, but sometimes crashing. Up and down, riding it in. Hopefully in control; frequently out of control. Feeling your own power and powers out of your control.

Midlife is certainly a time of transition. Transition from fertility to maturity. From youth to older age. There is no reason why life, if it's good, cannot continue to be good. And if it's crap—why it can't be modified or changed.

Nature (or fate) periodically provides windows of opportunity for us to take stock of both our physical and spiritual lives. For a woman, menopause is one of those windows which may either be a peep hole or a floor-to-ceiling vista, depending on attitude and circumstance.

Physical events in our bodies seem to repeat, coming and going. "Infancy" and "childhood" appear at both ends of our lives. So the irregularity and hecticity of the menstrual cycle in women's teens repeats, in unexpected ways, in her fourth and fifth decades. The wide swings in hormone levels and periodic anovulatory cycles (no ovulation) seen at ages 11-16, repeats at 40-55, leading to increases in "PMS" symptoms, fluid retention, and the non-synchronous bleeding episodes stemming from lack of ovulation. It is the "way of life."

An understanding of the normal physiology involved is helpful. Every female child is born with her full complement of immature oocytes or "eggs." Beginning usually in the earliest teens, several of these begin to mature each cycle and one or more "ovulate" each month in most women. As the egg matures and ovulates, the female hormones estrogen and progesterone are secreted into the blood stream and perform important functions as they travel throughout the body. Menarche (the beginning of ovulation and menstruation) sees the same wide up and down swings in hormonal output and irregular bleeding that accompany the menopause. It is almost the rule of previously "clockwork regular" women to experience, in their 40s, the occasional irregularity (two periods in a month, or missing a month altogether) and occasional days of spotting before or after menses which accompany the hormonal changes of impending menopause. (More frequent bleeding, especially without a pattern, might be cause for alarm and should lead to a visit to one's gynecologist.)

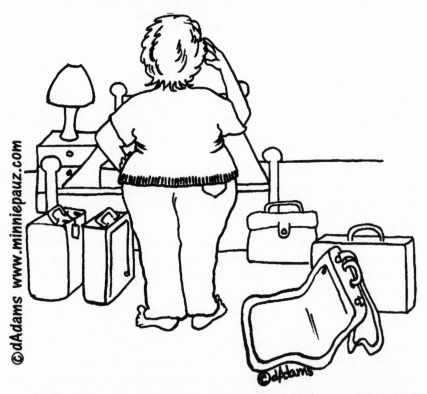

## I KNOW I was going somewhere, but WHERE?

Rather than looking with worry and alarm at these normal and physiological changes, the peri-menopausal years are a good time to take stock and to ask the question, "What do I want to be doing during the next 2-3 decades of my life?" It is certainly a time to assess diet, exercise routines, relationships and one's general level of health. It may be time to consider hormone replacement therapy (HRT) or other supplements. Although it is obvious that nature did not intend women to have any significant level of estrogen in their bodies after their 40s or 50s, there can be health and lifestyle benefits to be had from short-term HRT without sacrificing safety.

There are four phases related to menopause: <u>pre</u>-menopause, <u>peri</u>-menopause, menopause and <u>post</u>-menopause:

1. Pre-menopause is defined as the time between the first menstrual period and the last menstrual period and is referred to as "the reproductive years."
2. Peri-menopause is the time when a woman's body begins to change in preparation for menopause—the end of the child bearing years. Peri-menopause includes the several years prior to menopause and the first year after menopause. During this time, the ovary's production of hormones (estrogen, progesterone, and testosterone) decreases. As a result, uncomfortable experiences may occur, including hot flashes, vaginal dryness, urinary problems, mood changes, sleeplessness, lowered sexual desire, and difficulty concentrating. Cycles and periods may become shorter and lighter or longer and heavier, making bleeding patterns less predictable. Symptoms usually begin in the mid-40s but may begin as early as age 35. These symptoms can occur for 2-8 years, sometimes stopping when the menstrual periods end, sometimes taking years to subside. Women who have had ovaries surgically removed, or damaged as a result of cancer therapy ("induced menopause") may experience early (and severe) symptoms of menopause. Hysterectomy alone (without removal of ovaries) does <u>not</u> induce menopause.
3. Menopause is the final menstrual period. Menopause can only be known for sure by looking back a year or more after the event. The average age western women experience menopause is 50-51, but can occur anywhere from the late 30s to the late 50s.
4. Post-menopause is the phase of life that follows the final menstrual period.

Menopause is a natural biological event, not a disease or an "estrogen deficiency disease." Menopause happens to all women, but affects each one uniquely.

Many women traverse menopause with minimal discomfort during the peri-menopausal years. Usually disturbances diminish or disappear over time, or are reduced with lifestyle changes such as exercise and diet modification. Most disturbances decrease or disappear with treatment. As you will see elsewhere in this book, there are <u>many</u> different therapeutic modalities: hormonal (including bioidentical plant-sourced hormones), botanical, herbal, supplemental, psychoactive, and more. Many women need treatment of some sort and should not feel as if they have "failed" to manage menopause on their own. Each individual's unique makeup is different and unique treatment is required.

Not only is each woman unique, but therapeutic options keep changing. The information in this book is "state of the art," but research will continue to provide better guidelines, substances and delivery systems, so women can work with their health care providers to determine their individual health and health risk status to fashion a regimen to help them for years to come. It is so beneficial for a woman to take the time to work with a health care professional who is willing to <u>listen,</u> to determine special needs and recommend therapeutic adjustments as required as a woman's body continues to change in her own individual way.

## HEALTHCARE THROUGH MIDLIFE

Healthcare is just that. Caring for your health. Like investing $200 per month from age 18 will make you a millionaire by your mid-40s, caring daily for your health from a young age will go a long way towards assuring you healthy longevity.

We are just as likely, however, to care for our bodies appropriately in our <u>youth</u> as we are to begin investing as a teen. (No way!) "...If we only knew then what we do now..."

In our 40s (sometimes late 30s; for sure in our 50s), we KNOW we'd better get our act together if we want to live to play with our grandchildren—especially if we want to <u>enjoy</u> doing it.

We see the flab collecting. We have our first hot flash. Our pants don't get wet when we see Tom Cruise (in fact, we can't even fit into our pants). PMS raises its ugly head.

It is time to take charge.

Peri-menopause is an ideal time to begin or to reinforce a health promotion program that will serve you through the remainder of your life.

Since advancing age is happening anyway (Time marches on!), you might as well view midlife and menopause as the <u>beginning</u> of positive life and health changes.

## THE "ANNUAL CHECK UP"

Healthy behaviors and regular clinical exams are keys to health. Women of all ages, whether pre-menopausal, peri-menopausal or post-menopausal, benefit from an annual exam. As part of the checkup, various tests (blood, urine, saliva, ultrasound, x-ray, etc.) can be performed to further determine heart, bone, breast, pelvic and intestinal health. These tests can also help determine lipid/cholesterol levels and thyroid status. (Not infrequently, women become hypothyroid [low thyroid] at time of menopause, further diminishing energy reserves.) Most experts feel annual screening mammography (?? after age 40—for sure after age 50) is very beneficial in diagnosing breast cancer early—in fact, leading to the increased breast cancer survival being noticed in recent years.

Other tests (e.g., for diabetes, to help diagnose fatigue or urinary incontinence) can be performed as necessary. Hormone level measurements may be helpful, but are frequently misleading because hormonal levels can fluctuate, making testing unreliable.

During the checkup, key components to health can be discussed, including sexuality, exercise, smoking cessation, drug and alcohol use or abuse, physical abuse, stress reduction, improving sleep, attaining and maintaining ideal weight, ingesting sufficient calcium and other adequate nutrition, etc.

Various options can be discussed if needed. Alternative plans should include a discussion of risks and benefits and possible alternatives, a plan to watch for side effects, and a plan to monitor outcomes. Take nothing unless you know why you are taking it, what it is designed to accomplish, how it works, what side effects are possible, and which to expect on a short or long term basis. Make sure before you leave the office that a follow-up appointment has been scheduled within a reasonable (e.g., 6-12 weeks) length of time.

As women experience all of the (physical/emotional/social) changes of approaching menopause, they face a unique opportunity to develop their own strategies for midlife wellness. Each woman is an expert on her own body. As this expert, she (You!) will benefit more if you are well informed.

And that is the whole idea of this book: Information in one place, to better prepare and outfit you for your midlife passage.

*And hear the pleasant cuckoo, loud and long*
*The simple bird thinks two notes a song*
                              —W.H. Davies in *April's Charms*

# CHAPTER TWO

## ONE SIZE DOES NOT FIT ALL
### Finding the "Right Fit"; Dealing with Your Health Care Provider and Your Health Plan

The "one size fits all" concept that HMOs enforce on patient care doesn't quite fit many, if not most, women in their late 30s, 40s and 50s, most of whom are treated with the "take a test, give a pill" mentality necessitated by 10-minute office visits.

Midlife therapeutic options (for PMS, bleeding problems, symptom control, hormone therapy, pelvic support, etc., etc.) are a little like shopping for a good pair of shoes: one size DOES NOT fit all. That precisely is where managed care, with its "universal sizing" and "quick fits" fails midlife women. And that is the purpose of this book: to help you with the best possible fit. One that is comfortable, does not bind, wears well, and very importantly: LOOKS GOOD.

The approach of this book is a little like shopping for shoes at Nordstrom's or Saks. You come in needing a special pair of shoes. You have an idea as to what you want. There are a lot of shoes on the floor (and many more in the back room). You have a very knowledgeable sales person: (S)he will measure the exact size and shape of your foot and can suggest additional ideas to complement your original thoughts.

It may be the first pair you try...it may be the fifth. There is a style that works and a size that fits. You know you will walk out with a pair of shoes.

The plain fact is that there are so many viable midlife healthcare options; so many choices. The key is proper education, good knowledge (not myth) and understanding of the pros, cons, and applicability of all the different therapeutic options from estrogens and progestins to androgens and progesterone, from oral therapy to transdermals and compounded preparations, from botanicals to herbals.

A key here is self-awareness, the key word "empowerment." Can you sit down with yourself and consciously know and understand just what is happening right now? What you're concerned about. What you're scared of.

Where you'd like to be. How you'd like to get there. Fears, worries, concerns, desires, successes, failures. You must be able to verbalize these both to yourself and to your healthcare provider.

## "THE LIST"

...AND WRITE IT DOWN! When you see your healthcare provider, you may not need to refer to your "cheat sheet," but it's important to have it there, "for support." Just in case.

It is only through <u>knowing</u> yourself, your individual situation and needs, that you will be able to approach that personal nirvana known as <u>empowerment</u> in the areas of midlife comfort and healthcare.

This book will help you know yourself and, as importantly, know options available so that you can knowledgeably discuss (and demand) these with (and from) your health care provider. Well trained, intelligent, and secure healthcare providers welcome knowledgeable and prepared patients with whom they can share health care decisions.

Read and understand the chapters that pertain to your situation. If you wish, visit the appropriate web sites or read the wonderful specialized books listed in Chapter 20. Keep your mind open to as many ideas and avenues of therapy as possible. MAKE A LIST. Bring it in to your healthcare provider and work with him/her to fashion a therapy that fits your needs, with medications if possible that are in your healthcare plan formulary, although understanding that you <u>may</u> need to put out some extra bucks to get just the right "fit" for yourself—especially if a transdermal cream happens to work best for you (you don't want to get a blister just because the shoe is "on sale").

Also: make sure your practitioner makes a return appointment in at least ±3 months to <u>review and evaluate</u> how you are doing. Make this appointment when you leave. Do not wait 2-3 months or it might be 6 months before you are able to be seen again.

Make sure your practitioner discusses the usual happenings and side effects of your medications (especially those that are short-lived and will go away on their own). <u>Frequently</u> with a new therapy, it may seem as if it's not working or there are individual bothersome side effects...but usually all these "straighten themselves out" in a week or three. If you are unsure, don't just <u>quit</u> the medication: call your provider first!

If you have tried, but have not been able to get the "proper fit" from your primary care provider (even when armed with the ideas and knowledge gleaned from this book), how then do you proceed? (Remember, the definition of an HMO is an institution where patients are "sold to the <u>lowest</u> bidder!") It may then be appropriate for you to spend a few extra bucks to go "out of network" to a healthcare practitioner specializing in PMS or menopause.

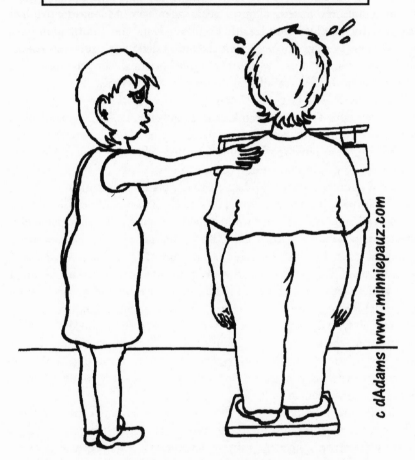

You're not heavy, you're my sister!

A useful resource for finding such a person in your geographic area is the North American Menopause Society's (NAMS) web site (http://www.menopause.org). On this site you can find the name and address of NAMS members in your area. The "best" are practitioners that have passed special examinations that qualify them as a "certified menopause clinician" (these certified practitioners' names are highlighted in the NAMS listings).

In 2000, a new measure, known as Management of Menopause (MOM) was added to HEDIS (the Health Employer Data and Information Set), which is a <u>performance management</u> tool, coordinated by a private, not-for-profit organization (the National Committee for Quality Assurance, or NCQA), established in 1990 and dedicated to improving the quality of healthcare in this country.

One of the NCQA's major activities is <u>accreditation</u> primarily of health plans. The HEDIS "report card," based on data submitted by participating health plans, appears in NCQA's "State of Managed Care Quality Report," which is published each fall and can be accessed on the Committee's website (http://www.ncqa.org). Check out how <u>your</u> health plan is doing, compared to others, especially in the area of MOM (Management of Menopause).

Additionally, the Jacobs Institute of Women's Health, an independent, non-profit organization that studies and disseminates information intended to advance the knowledge, practice, and understanding of women's healthcare, has developed a set of comprehensive guidelines aimed at health plans and practitioners. Copies of these "Guidelines for Counseling Women in the Management of Menopause" are available on the Institute's website (http://www.jiwh.org).

*"There must be some way out of here," said the joker to the thief*
*"There's too much confusion, I can't get no relief"*
—Bob Dylan in
*All Along the Watchtower*

# CHAPTER THREE

## PMS/PMDD
## The "Puppet on a String"

How does it feel to be a puppet on a string? To have your chain jerked by a puppet master outside of your control. To feel bloated, unable to fit into your clothes 1-2 weeks out of the month. To have your breasts so sore that you're ready to bite your son's or grandson's head off when he accidentally crashes into you.

PMS (Premenstrual Syndrome) is real! Now officially called PMDD (Premenstrual Dysphoric Disorder) if especially severe, it's a medical condition with a combination of emotional and physical symptoms which can disrupt health, career, and personal life.

Affecting as many as 80% of American women, this condition is often misunderstood or ignored. (Although if you're really suffering, it's tough to ignore it!) But the symptoms are real: premenstrual irritability, depression, bloating, headaches and weight gain, and carbohydrate craving are not all in the imagination.

But there is definitely hope for PMS/PMDD sufferers (as we will see below).

Some sort of premenstrual symptoms are common and, by definition, are a normal aspect of ovulatory cycles. Severe symptoms, however, that meet the official psychiatric criteria for PMDD are less common, occurring in approximately 5-10% of women.

Somewhere in between, however, are the many women whose symptoms are not severe enough for true psychiatric diagnosis, but bothersome enough nevertheless to warrant mitigation and therapy.

Advancing age is often cited as a risk factor for PMS/PMDD (most women seeking treatment are well over 30 years of age); however this syndrome can occur in menstruating women of any age. Genetics appear to play a role in some women with PMS/PMDD. There is no typical "personality profile" of women with PMS/PMDD. Premenstrual symptoms seem to affect women irrespective of cultural or socioeconomic status.

## WHAT CAUSES PMS?

Another $64,000 question! As they say medically: "The etiology of PMS is incompletely understood..." (translation: "We really don't know...").

It definitely appears that PMS is a "neuroendocrine disorder" involving the brain's sensitivity and reactivity to the circulating levels of hormones that course through it. In other words, especially in the peri-menopause, women's bodies respond in strange ways to the cyclic changes in their hormones (What else is new!). Thus, Drs. John Lee and Christiane Northrup's theory of "estrogen dominance" and its successful treatment with natural progesterone cream. Thus Drs. John Studd and Elizabeth Vliet's theories involving diminished estrogen levels[1] (the opposite of Drs. Lee and Northrup). I will explain these divergent views later.

Currently, the most plausible theory involves dysregulation (screwed up regulation) of serotonin, norepinephrine, dopamine and endorphins, the major brain chemicals that are involved in mood regulation. Thus the beneficial response to exercise (which increases endorphins, a brain chemical which serves to increase the amount of serotonin available) and to a class of medications known as SSRIs (selective serotonin reuptake inhibitors); e.g., Prozac®, Celexa®, etc., which increase the amount of serotonin on a constant basis, significantly improving the psychological PMS symptoms in a large percentage of women. (More about this later.)

## TYPICAL SYMPTOMS OF PMS

PMS symptoms vary in type, timing and severity from woman to woman, but typically begin during the two weeks before the period (premenstrually) and end after the period begins. Symptoms are of two types: emotional and physical, with difficult menses also a part of the equation.

---

[1]"New Perspectives on the Relationship of Hormone Changes to Affective Disorders in the Peri-menopause," E. L. Vliet, V. L. Hutcheson Davis, NACOG's Clinical Issues, 1991; 2:453-58.

Premenstrual syndrome and premenstrual Dysphoric Disorder, W. H. Cronje and J.W.W. Studd, Primary Care Clinics in Office Practice, 2002; 29:1-12.

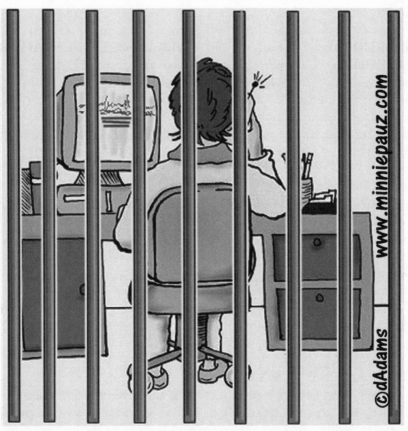

I don't know, the boss just mentioned something about
protecting the rest of the office on my "off" days.

## DO YOU HAVE PMS? TRY SCORING YOURSELF:

Grading of Symptoms:
0 = None
1 = Mild
2 = Moderate
3 = Severe/Disabling

| EMOTIONAL SYMPTOMS | WEEK BEFORE PERIOD | WEEK AFTER PERIOD |
|---|---|---|
| 1. Nervous Tension | 0 / 1 / 2 / 3 | 0 / 1 / 2 / 3 |
| 2. Mood Swings | 0 / 1 / 2 / 3 | 0 / 1 / 2 / 3 |
| 3. Irritability | 0 / 1 / 2 / 3 | 0 / 1 / 2 / 3 |
| 4. Depression | 0 / 1 / 2 / 3 | 0 / 1 / 2 / 3 |
| 5. Forgetfulness | 0 / 1 / 2 / 3 | 0 / 1 / 2 / 3 |
| 6. Anxiety | 0 / 1 / 2 / 3 | 0 / 1 / 2 / 3 |
| 7. Insomnia | 0 / 1 / 2 / 3 | 0 / 1 / 2 / 3 |
| 8. Crying/confusion | 0 / 1 / 2 / 3 | 0 / 1 / 2 / 3 |
| **PHYSICAL SYMPTOMS** | | |
| 1. Breast tenderness | 0 / 1 / 2 / 3 | 0 / 1 / 2 / 3 |
| 2. Abdominal Bloating | 0 / 1 / 2 / 3 | 0 / 1 / 2 / 3 |
| 3. Weight gain | 0 / 1 / 2 / 3 | 0 / 1 / 2 / 3 |
| 4. Craving for Sweets | 0 / 1 / 2 / 3 | 0 / 1 / 2 / 3 |
| 5. Headache | 0 / 1 / 2 / 3 | 0 / 1 / 2 / 3 |
| 6. Increased appetite | 0 / 1 / 2 / 3 | 0 / 1 / 2 / 3 |
| 7. Menstrual cramps/pain/heavy flow | 0 / 1 / 2 / 3 | 0 / 1 / 2 / 3 |

The higher you score for the "week before period," especially if it is 15 or more, the more likely you have PMS/PMDD, which may be interfering with your life. If your score for the "week after period" is also high, what you have may not be PMS, but primarily a psychological situation which may be best helped by psychotherapy and/or medication.

LET'S UNDERSTAND WHAT'S GOING ON

Everyone, male or female, responds to their environment. If your environment (e.g., driving in dense traffic, dealing with an unreasonable boss, staining your best blouse) has produced a stressful day, you may react more stridently than usual when your son whines that he can't get his shoe tied. What is a more intimate part of a woman's environment than her hormones/hormonal levels? These intimate actions and interactions can combine to produce some quite disconcerting symptoms (as noted above).

## THE SEROTONIN CONNECTION AND THE SLEEP CYCLE

Serotonin is a brain chemical produced from L-Tryptophan, an essential amino acid (or nutritional "building block") found in many foods. Some people don't produce enough serotonin, which may interfere with sleep, the menstrual cycle, or carbohydrate metabolism.

Serotonin helps you sleep well. Low serotonin may produce abnormal sleep, which helps produce the emotional symptoms of PMS.

Additionally, serotonin helps regulate menstrual hormones. Low serotonin may cause early ovulating, an imbalance of estrogen and progesterone, and the physical symptoms of PMS.

Serotonin also helps regulate appetite; low serotonin may create food cravings, especially for sweets and other carbohydrates.

The low levels of serotonin common in women with PMS/PMDD may affect the amount and quality of sleep, especially prior to menstruation. A normal sleep cycle produces plenty of quality REM ("rapid eye movement") sleep, the stage during which dreaming occurs. Poor/abnormal sleep, frequently found in women (and men) with low serotonin levels, with little time in REM and frequent wake-ups, produces or exacerbates most of the emotional symptoms related to PMS/PMDD. Irritability, anger, depression, fatigue, confusion, tension, anxiety and inability to concentrate are all connected with poor sleep quality.

## THE HORMONAL CONNECTION

The menstrual cycle is a complex and often delicate hormonal balance. Many things: abnormal levels of serotonin and other brain chemicals, abnormal development of the egg follicles, etc., may throw off the timing and quality of ovarian hormones and ovulation, thus affecting hormonal balance. These hormonal changes seem to be responsible for the physical symptoms associated with PMS.

In the normal menstrual cycle, serotonin and hormonal interactions suppress LH (leutenizing hormone), the hormone responsible for ovulation. At ± day 13-15 of the menstrual cycle, this hormone surges, causing ovulation to occur. During the second half of the cycle, estrogen and progesterone are "in balance" and PMS symptoms do not occur, or are minimal.

In abnormal cycles, especially frequent at midlife, serotonin levels may be too low to suppress LH, or for other reasons it "surges" too soon, triggering too-early ovulation. This may lead to a lowered progesterone level and a relative excess of estrogen. As or more frequently perhaps, the mood disorders and fluid retention seen are a response to <u>lowered</u> level of estrogens in relation to progesterone, or co-existing <u>with</u> a low progesterone. These imbalances cause the physical symptoms of PMS/PMDD (tender breasts, bloating, weight gain, constipation followed by diarrhea, and occasional acne).

## CARBOHYDRATE METABOLISM

Serotonin levels also help control carbohydrate metabolism and food cravings. When serotonin levels are low, you may crave too much carbohydrate (especially refined carbohydrates such as sugar and chocolate). The body seems to be trying to increase serotonin by eating carbohydrates which help the brain absorb L-Tryptophan, the amino acid needed to make serotonin.

## DEVELOPING A TREATMENT PROTOCOL THAT WILL WORK FOR YOU

In order to fashion a program which works for you, you first need to be aware of the problems. Is it the emotional symptoms (tension, anxiety, irritability, etc.), the physical symptoms (bloating, breast tenderness, etc.) or the menstrual cramping that predominates; or a combination of factors? Different approaches are used for the different symptoms, although they certainly can be combined. And The mainstays of therapy, diet and exercise, are discussed below. Check your score on the PMS symptoms questionnaire to see which type (types) of symptoms you are treating.

The two mainstays of PMS/PMDD treatment are diet and exercise (sorry, there's no "free lunch"). Like so many other things discussed in this book, there are few magic bullets. You need to do the basic work, the building blocks, yourself before medications and other modifications can kick in and help. Good nutrition, sleep and stress management, and exercise all seem to help raise serotonin levels (the key), which will help reduce your symptoms.

## PMS TREATMENT PROGRAM OUTLINE

I.  For everybody: General Measures
    A.  Nutrition and Exercise Program
        1. Caffeine Reduction: If you are a "chocaholic" or heavy coffee/tea/cola drinker, start reducing caffeine at all times (make your coffee "half-caf" by mixing half regular, half decaf; substitute decaf sodas, etc.) so that when you need to stop caffeine at PMS times, it won't be so much of a shock to your system.
        2. Healthy Diet: Low-fat, salt, sugar, processed foods. If it comes in a can, a jar, or if you have to peel off a wrapper: forget it! Alcohol

and especially caffeine are "death" to PMS sufferers (if it's a "brown liquid," don't drink it). Avoid artificial sweeteners (they interfere with L-Tryptophan, an essential amino acid). Eat mostly "complex" carbohydrates (whole grains, fruits, vegetables). A diet high in these will help L-Tryptophan reach the brain and will improve sleep.

3. <u>Exercise</u>: Helps reduce symptoms in two ways. (1) it's a stress reducer, so it helps you sleep better; (2) <u>vigorous</u>, sweaty, "out of breath" exercise produces endorphins in the brain. Endorphins, in turn, raise the brain's serotonin levels naturally, helping alleviate PMS. Whatever the exercise program that you usually engage in, if you really want to FEEL BETTER, and not "PMS so much," you <u>must</u> get at least 20-30 minutes (40-50 is better) of <u>sweaty, out of breath, heart pumping</u> (e.g., fast walking, running, aerobics, fast sports, etc.) exercise <u>each</u> day during the last 7-14 days of your menstrual cycle.

4. Vitamin and mineral supplements also help raise serotonin levels. Especially helpful are vitamins B6 (approximately 100 mg per day), vitamin E (400-800 I.U. per day), and a calcium/magnesium supplement (~1000/500 mg). Evening Primrose oil and/or chaste berry/chaste fruit extract are also helpful in relieving symptoms.

B. <u>"Sleep Hygiene" Program</u>: Sleep quality and quantity can be an important factor in alleviating PMS symptoms. Try to get at least 8 hours of uninterrupted sleep each night—more after mid-cycle. How can you do this?

1. Arrange a comfortable sleep environment. Keep your room dark and quiet, with shades and drapery; use ear plugs and an eye mask, if necessary.

2. Sleep consistent hours; take naps and rest breaks to supplement, if necessary.

3. Follow a bedtime routine or bedtime ritual (see Chapter 13).

4. Explain the importance of sleep in improving your mood to your family so that they can be quieter in the morning, making their own breakfast, etc. ("Would you rather have me make breakfast, or not bite your head off in the morning?" might be a good opener.)

II. <u>For Pre-menstrual Physical and Emotional Symptoms</u>

A. Vitamin E 400-800 I.U. per day may help with breast tenderness.

B. **Hormones**

Estrogen. You can try this "on spec" or, more scientifically, by either blood or salivary testing, 2-4 times in the last 7 days of two menstrual cycles.

If estrogen level is low, or low-normal, and progesterone levels are fine, try low-mid dose estrogen supplementation with a patch or pill. If levels of <u>both</u> estrogen and progesterone are low, you may want to try both hormones. Some people even feel that adding a bit of testosterone helps, especially for loss of energy and loss of libido.

<u>Progesterone cream</u>. Although the science is a bit soft, natural progesterone cream (derived usually from wild Mexican yam root) has staunch and articulate allies in John Lee, M.D., and Christiane Northrup, M.D., and seems to help frequently with PMS symptoms of bloating, breast tenderness, and some of the emotional symptoms as well. The usual dosage is approximately ¼ tsp. (measure it out at first with a ¼ tsp. measuring spoon and then scoop it out of the spoon with your little finger—after a short time, you will be able to estimate it directly from the jar. (It's not "rocket science"; the dose doesn't need to be exact.) The cream is massaged into the soft skin of the underside of your inner arm or inner thigh, usually at bedtime.

Progesterone cream can be found at most health food and large drug stores, but which kind do you get? The strongest is the best. Try to get 3-5% cream (look for the numbers "3" or "5," if dosage is discussed on the label, or "3 gms per oz...5 gms per oz."). Avoid creams with no dosage given. The progesterone in these creams is a "bioidentical," synthesized, using Mexican yam root, to mimic the chemical structure of human progesterone. The best way is to get a 3-5% cream or gel (use 50-150 mg each evening) made up by a <u>compounding pharmacist</u> (see Chapter 7).

Drs. Lee & Northrup feel progesterone is the thing. Drs. Studd and Vliet (with perhaps more science behind them) feel that progesterone <u>causes</u> PMS-like symptoms, and suggest estrogen.

The importance is individualization. I wish I could give a PMS recipe that would help for everyone. Doesn't work that way, unfortunately. But—hormone additions to provide stabilization usually help. (The question is: which <u>one</u>—or <u>both</u>??)

C. If water retention and bloating remain a problem, diuretics ("water pills"), prescribed by your doctor, may help. In extreme cases of estrogen dominance, an "estrogen level reducer medication" (danocrine or Danazol® at low doses of 100-200 mg per day during the last 10-14 days of the cycle) may help do the job.

D. Specifically for emotional symptoms: If you are really bothered by PMS, and if you really want to do something about it, and thus are religious about following the nutritional and exercise guidelines perhaps with the correct supplemental hormone therapy, you will find, after a short time (2-3 months) that your symptoms definitely will improve. But understand also, PMS is chronic, will probably be with you until menopause, and will wax and wane. If the nutritional and exercise regimens do not alleviate your symptoms sufficiently, there is another important and frequently excellent medical therapy available that can be prescribed by your doctor.

There is a class of medications known as "SSRIs" (selective serotonin reuptake inhibitors), which inhibit the reuptake (or removal) of serotonin from the brain. Translation: they increase the amount of serotonin available in the brain. It used to be thought that these medications [fluoxetine ("Prozac®"), serataline ("Zoloft®") citralopam ("Celexa®"), paroxetine ("Paxil®") and the newly available "Lexapro®"] had to be taken on a day-in, day-out basis to be effective, but we know now that they may be taken in low doses (e.g., 10-20 mg per day for Prozac® or Celexa®) during PMS-times only (e.g., the last 10-14 days of the cycle) and can give relief for the emotional symptoms of PMS.

III. For "The Period": PMS/PMDD sufferers frequently have difficult menses as well, with significant cramps and heavier than normal bleeding. A good first-line therapy here is the addition of 600 mg of ibuprofen (3 over the counter tablets) 3 times a day, or 450 mg of Naprosin (2 over the counter tablets of Aleve®) twice a day, both taken with meals or food, starting 2-3 days before the expected period and continuing through the days of heavy flow.

If this is insufficient, "birth control pill cycling" frequently helps with these symptoms.

Important to Note: If you are "freaking out" with some regularity, it's nice to have a "panic pill" at your disposal ("what to do till the doctor comes"). Alprazolam ("Xanax®") doesn't cure your PMS (you will go a long ways toward doing that by following the outline above—then you probably won't need the Xanax®), but it sure helps maintain equilibrium if severe anxiety, stress, tension and basically being "out of control" is part of your equation. If you need, ask your doc to write a small prescription for the 0.5 mg dosage. You'll probably only need ½ the dosage (0.25 mg) but occasionally the full 0.5 mg is necessary and it's more cost-effective to take one half of the higher dose. But remember: Alprazolam (Xanax®) is habit-forming, so do not rely on it for anything other than a "fallback," taken occasionally as needed.

Menstrual Migraine

This is as good a time as any to discuss menstrual migraine. Migraine headaches can strike anyone at any time, but are more common in women than in men and tend to occur with increased frequency and severity as women mature through late reproductive and peri-menopausal years. It is well known that there are hormonal relationships to migraine headaches.

Birth control pills may make them worse—or better. Likewise, pregnancy can do away with, or intensify, migraine.

Menstrual migraine is the phenomenon, familiar to many migraine sufferers, of regular, cyclic intensification of their migraine on the day before, during, and just after their menses.

There is a clear physiologic explanation for this. Hormonal estradiol levels wax and wane during the menstrual cycle, with minor variations from cycle-to-cycle during reproductive years. Estrogen is lowest, however, in the day(s) prior to, during, and the day or two after the menses, rising again as the egg follicles begin to mature.

Thus, menstrual migraines occur, or are clearly intensified by the fall from the estradiol levels the body was used to during the preceding few weeks.

The problem is intensified during the late reproductive and peri-menopausal years, when these hormonal swings intensify, leading often to higher highs and therefore comparatively lower lows.

What to do?? If this is the pattern of your migraine (occurring more frequently or intensifying during this period of time), ask your health care practitioner to try a mid-dose estrogen supplementation for approximately 1 week, beginning ± one day before your expected cyclic "bad days."

This can be with oral estradiol (0.5-1 mg per day) or conjugated estrogen (0.3-0.625 mg per day). An alternate way is to apply an estradiol patch, ±0.05 mg, either Climera®, which lasts for 7 days, or one of the other 3-4 day patches (Vivelle®, Alora®, Esclim®, etc.), applying a second patch four days after the first.

If you are on oral contraceptives, try Mircette®, which contains a small amount of estrogen (but no progestin, so you still will have your period) during 5 of the 7 "placebo days."

Another key to migraine protection is prompt action. At the first little hint of headache, promptly take ibuprofen 600 mg with food, or a tablet of

Fiorinal®. The key is promptness! The worst thing that can happen is that you might take these rather benign medications occasionally when you might not need them. Important also is to have some Imitrex®, Maxalt®, etc., on hand, should the nasty monster take hold.

## PMS THERAPEUTIC FLOW SHEET

| For Emotional Symptoms | | For Both | For Physical Symptoms |
|---|---|---|---|
| **FIRST TIER** | Alprazolam (Xanax®) as needed, initially | 1. Dietary modification: Avoid caffeine, simple sugars, alcohol. Favor complex carbohydrates (grains, fresh fruit, vegetables, pasta, etc.)<br>2. Do daily exercise<br>3. Stress/sleep management; Do bedtime ritual w/sleep aids (Valerian, Kava, etc.) as needed.<br>4. Progesterone cream and/or estrogen, in form of a patch. | Vitamin E and progesterone cream and/or estrogen |
| **SECOND TIER** | Add-in SSRI (Celexa®, Prozac®, Paxil®, Zoloft®, etc.) | Vitamin/Herbal Therapy: Vitamin $B_6$, Calcium and magnesium. Herbs such as evening primrose oil, chaste berry extract. | Diuretics ("water pills") – hydrochlorothiazide, spironolactone |
| **THIRD TIER** | Explore biofeedback, psychotherapy, behavioral therapy, relaxation therapy, chiropractic, and massage | Try oral contraceptive cycling<br><br>Try Bromocryptine | Add-in anti-estrogen such as danocrine (Danazol®) |

## SALLY'S STORY

Sally came into my office self-described as "in pretty good shape, all things considered..." "I'm here at a good time," she confided. "I've just finished my period. You should have seen me last week." I responded that it was just as well, as I charged PMS patients extra when they came in during their "bad weeks." We both agreed that that probably would be the *coup de grace* for someone who was "PMSing real bad," and we got down to business.

Sally was fairly typical for the community in which I practice. With one pre-teen son, and a teen-aged daughter, she also taught 5th grade at Pioneer Elementary. I commented that she had a pretty full plate, but she assured me that she enjoyed the dual roles and had always handled things quite well until the past year or two.

"I've always had a bit of PMS," she told me. "I could always tell when my period was coming; I'd get bloated and my breasts would get tender for a few days before my period, and I'd be a bit grouchy: nothing I couldn't handle. But beginning last year, or the year before...maybe it was my 40th birthday, I don't know...I really began noticing a change. Instead of just a few days, which I could handle, I began to feel bad for more than a week. And it wasn't just being bloated and tender (although I wouldn't let my husband touch me during this time). I noticed myself getting so short-tempered and snapping at my students. When a couple of the boys in my class were teasing a girl during recess, I way overreacted and almost slapped one of them. At home, I find I'm countering my 14-year-old daughters' high drama with my own. It's like I'm no longer in control of myself for almost 2 weeks a month. And my menstrual cramps have gotten so bad...it's like I only have 1-2 good weeks a month!"

I asked Sally what she wanted to accomplish. She responded, "To feel I have some control over my own life, despite what my cycle does."

I inquired regarding diet and exercise. "I used to work out at the gym 4-5 times a week," she told me. "But since Rima started gymnastics and Kyle is playing middle school sports, with all the chauffeuring I've hardly had the chance." Her diet was a bit haphazard, reflecting her hectic schedule. She only had one cup of coffee a day, "But it's Peet's," she said, naming a premium high-caf dark roast blend. However, she admitted that she drank up to 3-4 glasses of iced tea daily, and enjoyed a glass or two of wine with supper.

We started by having Sally fill out an MSQ, a "menstrual symptoms questionnaire," to have an objective measure with which to plan and follow treatment. I also checked blood levels of both estrogen and progesterone near the end of her cycle.

For the first tier of therapy, we started with diet and exercise. I asked Sally to begin drinking "half-caf" coffee (a mixture of one half regular, one half decaf), going to decaf only during PMS times. In addition, she was to substitute herbal tea for at least one half of her iced tea consumption (more if possible during PMS times). She began taking a high B/high C multivitamin, with calcium and magnesium, plus vitamin E 800 mg a day during PMS times.

Most importantly, we instituted an exercise routine. I explained to her that she shouldn't look on exercise as something she should like, but something she must do, if she wanted to feel better and stay fit in the bargain. I even wrote her an official prescription for "30-45 minutes of vigorous, sweaty, out of breath exercise, q.d. (every day)." "Don't look on exercise as fun," I told her. "Look on it as work, something you must do and at least (if not more) important than your other jobs, such as work, housekeeping, chauffeuring, etc. Put it at the top of your list," I told her. "It will make the other chores easier."

To aid in sleep quality, Sally began a modified bedtime ritual (see Chapter 13), setting aside 20 minutes (10-minute warm bath with an herbal tea drink, plus 10-minute breath meditation), which she subtracted from her sleep time (She was to find out that this investment was to be rewarded with better sleep quality and she told me later that she expanded it to 30, then 45 minutes ("instead of watching TV").

Since her progesterone level seemed to be falling late in her cycle (and because she brought it up, I won't discount the placebo effect), I asked Sally to use approximately ¼-½ tsp. of progesterone cream (she had found a 3% cream at her pharmacy) at bedtime, beginning day 15 of her cycle and ending with the onset of menses. (Sally initially started using the cream in the morning, but noticed that it made her drowsy, so she switched to bedtime.)

I offered Sally a small prescription for alprazolam (Xanax®) as a "back-up," which she refused.

We continued with this regimen for 2½ months, when Sally returned for follow-up. She had been keeping an MSQ. Where her total score was 28 before treatment, she had dropped to a total of 14. Although improved, she still complained of more breast tenderness and heavier, crampier menses than she'd like. Emotionally, "although not perfect," she was able to cope and specifically noted that she felt more rested when she got up in the morning.

I re-examined her, and performed an endovaginal pelvic ultrasound to recheck the uterus for any sign of fibroid or polyp, which I did not find. We added in some ibuprofen, 600 mg (3 of the over the counter generics),

3 times a day with meals, starting when she felt her period was "around the corner" and continuing the ibuprofen through heavy flow. Additionally, I started her on a low dose (100 mg per day) of danocrine hydrochloride (Danazol®), an "anti-estrogen," used in much higher doses for endometriosis. This, I explained, would slightly lower her estrogen levels in the last part of the cycle, hopefully helping with the mastalgia (breast tenderness). Additionally, I hoped it would lessen the amount of uterine lining (endometrium) and, along with the elevated tissue levels of ibuprofen she would be developing, would decrease the amount of her menstrual flow and cramps.

Two months later, Sally's scores were 8 and 10 (not too dissimilar to her scoring the week after the menses). She still felt a bit edgy during the week prior to her menses. I offered her a trial of one of the SSRI medications, but she didn't feel it to be necessary and felt her life to be back under her control. She was even "meditating" 15-20 minutes in the morning before breakfast and her daughter had even joined her. "She was sure I was on some sort of drugs," Sally told me. "One day when she saw me 'sitting,' she just popped down beside me and she's joined me more or less since."

*There were times when it seemed to [her] that the different parts of [her] were not all under the same management*
—Russell Hoban, from
*The Lion of Boaz-Jachin and Jachin-Boaz*

# CHAPTER FOUR

## BLEEDING PROBLEMS
### "But I <u>used</u> to be regular"

The only thing "normal" or "regular" about a woman's menstrual cycle is that it is not regular. Sure, many, if not most, women have a fairly reliable, more or less "regular" menstrual cycle in their 20s and 30s, but so many things (emotional factors, physical factors, and hormonal factors) can so easily throw it off.

Women with irregular cycles are less bothered by the typical pre- and peri-menopausal menstrual cyclic changes than are women who were previously "clockwork regular."

Approaching the late 30s and 40s, cycles can be longer, shorter, heavier, lighter, crampier, or less painful. Both "extra periods" and "missed periods" are common.

During the reproductive years, two of the hormones made by the ovaries, estrogen and progesterone, play important roles in the menstrual cycle. Estrogen, secreted by the cells surrounding the developing egg follicles causes the endometrium (lining of the uterus) to thicken in preparation for egg implantation. Progesterone, secreted from the ovary after ovulation, then causes a ripening of this tissue to support a possibly implanted egg.

If a fertilized egg is not received into the uterus, the ovaries stop making these hormones and the uterine lining is shed as the menstrual period ("the weeping of a disappointed endometrium"). Each woman's pattern is slightly different.

Around time of menopause, some women simply stop menstruating one day and never have another period. Most women, however, go through a longer peri-menopause and have changes and irregularities in their periods caused by erratic secretion of ovarian hormones and frequently associated with lack of ovulation or irregular ovulation and changes in the pattern and levels of ovarian hormone release. Usually a woman's cycle will get shorter;

menstrual bleeding may be shorter or heavier, less or more days. Skipping periods frequently occurs. Some women skip several cycles and then for a time menstruate regularly again. Any menstrual pattern is possible: what is noticeable is the change.

For most women, these changes are natural and normal during peri-menopause and no therapy is necessary.

## HOW DO YOU KNOW IF YOUR PATTERN IS ABNORMAL?

When should you seek therapy? The following bleeding patterns should generate a visit to your health care provider:

* Periods that are persistently heavy, "gushing," or accompanied by clots larger than your finger.
* Periods lasting over 7 days (or 2-3 days longer than usual).
* Regular spotting or bleeding happening in between menses, or irregular bleeding/spotting without a pattern.
* Intervals regularly shorter than 21 days from the start of one menses to the start of the next.
* Vaginal bleeding after lovemaking (occurring more than once or twice).

## POSSIBLE CAUSES OF ABNORMAL PERI-MENOPAUSAL BLEEDING INCLUDE:

1. Hormonal imbalance between levels of estrogen and progesterone, frequently caused by skipping ovulation or by the ripening of less (or more) eggs than usual.
2. Imbalance in thyroid hormone levels. Peri-menopause is a common time for a thyroid abnormality to manifest itself. The thyroid gland is part of the energy regulatory system of the body; however, abnormally high or (usually) a low level of secretion can effect the menstrual pattern.
3. Pregnancy. Remember, until menopause is reached pregnancy can occur and cause abnormal bleeding and/or missed periods.
4. Abnormalities of the uterine lining (endometrium). Non-cancerous growths such as polyps and pseudopolyps or hyperplasia (too much growth) in the endometrium can cause abnormal uterine bleeding.
5. Fibroids. Fibroids are benign (999 times out of 1000) muscle growths within or on the uterus and are frequently responsible for abnormal uterine bleeding. Their symptoms depend more on their location than their size. However, independent of location, they usually cause symptoms if they get large. Fibroids within the uterus can frequently cause irregular bleeding; those within the muscle of the uterus cause heavy/crampy/flooding menses and frequently backache pain. Growths on the surface of the uterus can cause pain, pressure and difficulties with

urination or bowel movements. While the cause of fibroids is unknown (they are benign tumors of the muscle of the uterus) their growth is stimulated by the estrogen surges that sometimes occur during peri-menopause. Fibroids usually shrink and their symptoms dissipate after menopause when the ovaries reduce their production of estrogen. Post menopausal hormone replacement therapy can occasionally stimulate fibroids but rarely does so as the amount of estrogen in hormone replacement therapy is but a fraction of that produced by even peri-menopausal ovaries.

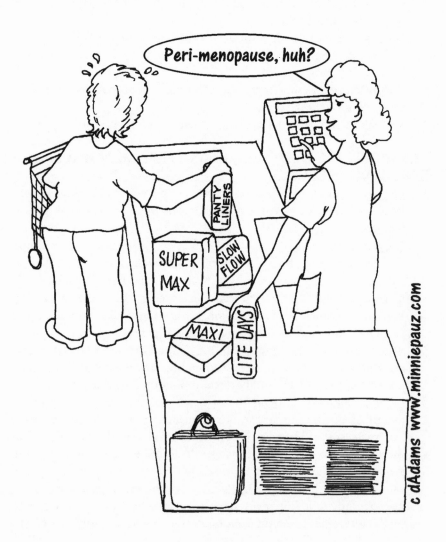

6.   Ovarian cysts. Frequently an ovarian cyst (invariably transient and benign) will cause an abnormal bleeding pattern. These are well diagnosed and followed by endovaginal pelvic ultrasound (ultrasound of the pelvis done by means of a vaginally-applied probe-see below). They rarely require any significant therapy and usually go away on their own.

7.   Cancer. In a very small percentage of cases, abnormal bleeding is caused by a uterine or, more rarely, vaginal or ovarian malignancy. Regular pelvic exams and Pap smears are helpful in diagnosis of these diseases early enough for effective treatment.

8.   Other causes of abnormal peri-menopausal bleeding include blood clotting problems and, rarely, other abnormalities in the vagina or cervix.

## DIAGNOSING THE CAUSE

If you have what you or your health care provider feels is abnormal uterine bleeding, before it can be properly treated the cause must be made known. There are several procedures to aid in this search:

1.   Endovaginal pelvic ultrasound (EVUS). This painless, non-invasive procedure utilizes sound-generated images (same as the procedure used during pregnancy), to produce a 2-dimensional image of the body of the uterus, the uterine cavity and ovaries. The very best way is for your health care provider her/himself to do the ultrasound in the office at the time of your visit. If your provider is not trained, or does not have access to an ultrasound machine and "orders" an ultrasound to be done in the radiology department, make sure that you look at the requisition slip. Has your provider written specifically what he/she wants looked at and described?? The information gained from the procedure (and written by the radiologist on his/her report) will only be as good as the images taken by the technician and then interpreted by the radiologist who "reads" the film later. If the technologist or radiologist do not know what your provider is specifically looking for, they might not look closely enough, and miss something.

2.   Sonohysterography. In this variation of ultrasound, a liquid is infused into the uterus, enhancing (by contrast) visualization of abnormalities within the uterine cavity. It is the "next best thing to being there" (see hysteroscopy, below).

3.   Endometrial biopsy. This widely used procedure, performed in the clinician's office usually without anesthesia, obtains random small samples of the uterine lining, which is then interpreted by a pathologist. It can be helpful in establishing a diagnosis especially if, on ultrasound

or sonohysterography, the abnormal process in the uterus appears to be more widespread than small and specific (like a polyp or fibroid). However, since it is a relatively "blind" procedure, if your problem persists, sonohysterography (see above) and/or hysteroscopy (see below) should be performed for more accurate information. If your problem persists even if you have had a "negative" endometrial biopsy, you must proceed with a more accurate diagnostic investigation. Especially if you are in a health care plan and have abnormal bleeding but have had a "negative" biopsy, don't let your practitioner tell you, "Don't worry, because your biopsy was normal." Have it investigated further.

4. Hysteroscopy. This is the "gold standard" of diagnostic procedures for abnormal uterine bleeding in which, usually under a local anesthetic, a clinician can actually look at the entire uterine lining with a special telescope called a "hysteroscope." If an abnormality is visualized, frequently it can be biopsied or removed at the same time (although sometimes this requires more extensive surgery and is performed at a later date).

## THERAPEUTIC OPTIONS

I. Hormone Therapy

When the abnormal uterine bleeding is caused by alterations in the usual internal hormonal interrelationships, it can often be regulated with prescription hormones.

The choices are:

1. Estrogen alone: Rarely used for abnormal bleeding problems; estrogen alone is used to help with other peri-menopausal symptoms (see next chapter).

2. Progesterone alone: Frequently progesterone alone, usually in the form of a long-used and safe artificial progesterone (or "progestin") called "Provera®" (generic: medroxyprogesterone acetate or MPA), is utilized to control irregular bleeding patterns caused by lack of ovulation or abnormal ovulation, especially when there is prolonged spotting. This is often used first, as a so-called "therapeutic trial" even before diagnostic studies. (If it works, other diagnostic studies may not be necessary.) "Provera®" works approximately 50% of the time. If it does, fine. If not (give it at least a couple of months), return to your physician.

(Note: Around 5-10% of women are psychologically quite sensitive to Provera®, noticing depression, tension, stress and generally feeling "yucky" on it. If this is the case, notify your health care provider so that (s)he can change therapy.)

3.  Estrogen and progesterone in combination: Usually given as a low-dose birth control pill, patch or vaginal ring, this pre-packaged form of estrogen and progesterone often has the perfect hormonal balance to manage the irregular bleeding patterns of the peri-menopause while additionally providing contraception and frequently helping with other disturbing peri-menopausal symptoms (see next chapter). However, as much as these can be helpful, cigarette smokers or women with varicose veins or liver problems are not candidates, and some women have side effects that preclude their usage. These may include adverse psychological symptoms, fluid retention and diminished sexual desire.

    If diminished libido is part of what's going on with you, oral contraceptives may not be the best therapy, as they, like all oral forms of replacement estrogen increase a blood protein called "sex hormone binding globulin" (SHBG). SHBG binds (or removes from circulation) free testosterone, further lowering the already low testosterone levels in peri-menopausal women. This can lead to a further lowering of libido. If this is the case, try the birth control patch (OrthoEvra®) or ring (Nuvaring®).

    A new and excellent non-surgical option for heavy menses (after diagnostic procedures have ruled out polyp or tumor) is to have the new IUD, "Mirena®," inserted. In addition to providing contraception if needed, it is very effective (after 1-2 months) in dramatically cutting down bleeding. It does this by means of a long-acting time release progestin (levonorgestrol) implanted within the small device.

II.  Non-Hormonal Medications

    Occasionally, heavy crampy periods can be controlled with a combination of non-steroidal anti-inflammatory drugs (NSAIDs), e.g., naproxen ("Naprosyn®"), ibuprofen, etc., and/or vitamins, as well as "anti-fibrinolytic agents." The latter, only occasionally used, are medications which enable the blood to clot better, sometimes diminishing heavy flow.

    Something that works for some people (and is safe) that you can try is to use ibuprofen ("Advil®") 600 mg (3 over-the-counter tablets) three times a day with food, or naproxen ("Aleve®") 440 mg (2 over-the-counter tablets) two times a day with food. Start this medication 2-3 days before your expected menses and continue through the heavy flow. Additionally, if you wish, add vitamin A 10,000 I.U. twice daily during these days. Give this regimen 2-3 months to see if it helps with heavy flow and cramps.

III. Surgical Options

   If these non-surgical treatments fail, several surgical procedures are available, depending on the cause of the abnormal bleeding. These include:

1.  D&C. Used more in past years (for both diagnosis and therapy of abnormal bleeding) than presently, it is a relatively blind procedure wherein a curette (like a tiny, hollow spoon) is used to clean (euphemism for "scrape") the inner lining of the uterus. It may or may not cure the abnormal bleeding, but is a good (but invasive) diagnostic procedure. Performed under local anesthesia with sedation, or general anesthetic.

2.  Operative Hysteroscopy. Presently the "gold standard" of diagnostic and therapeutic procedures in which a telescope is inserted into the uterus and the surgeon can directly see the entire uterine cavity and biopsy or otherwise treat as needed. Polyps, fibroids and excessive tissue can be cauterized or removed as indicated. Performed under either local or general anesthesia.

3.  Endometrial Ablation. In this procedure, the basal "generating" layer of the uterine lining is destroyed by heating, freezing, "radio waves," laser or cauterization. A good procedure for excessive, heavy menses in the absence of fibroids, it "cures" the problem either by stopping periods altogether or making them light and manageable in over 80% of patients. Occasionally, it needs to be repeated. Performed under local anesthesia with sedation or general anesthetic.

4.  Laparoscopy. In which a slender telescope, inserted through the naval, can very accurately view the entire pelvis and most of the abdominal cavity. Frequently, fibroids or ovarian cysts, etc., can be removed as necessary. Usually performed under a general anesthetic.

5.  Abdominal or Laparoscopic Myomectomy. Either through the 'scope or via an abdominal incision, fibroids that are causing pain or abnormal bleeding can be removed. There is no reason to do this procedure unless the patient desires to retain her uterus and preserve fertility. Performed under a general anesthetic.

6.  Uterine Artery Embolization. Small foam particles or "plastic beads" are instilled by a specially-trained radiologist into the uterine artery to block blood flow to fibroids, causing them to shrink. This is a very new procedure and may be a good alternative to surgery in women who cannot or do not want to undergo surgery and desire to retain their uterus. It is usually performed on an outpatient basis, although the initial 2-3 days of recovery is frequently quite painful.

7. <u>Laparoscopic or vaginal uterine artery ligation; myolysis</u>. Both "conservative, uterus-sparing procedures for fibroids. In the former, the uterine arteries are "tied" or cauterized. In myolysis, special fork-like probes are pushed into the fibroid to help destroy it. Both procedures (for women with symptomatic fibroids who wish to retain their uterus) should be performed by advanced laparoscopists only.

8. <u>Hysterectomy (abdominal, vaginal, laparoscopically assisted)</u>. Over 50% of hysterectomies in the United States are performed for fibroids and/or abnormal bleeding. The uterus (and frequently the cervix also) is removed. The ovaries may or may not be removed (called "oophorectomy" if ovary is removed). If both ovaries are removed ("bilateral oophorectomy"), immediate "surgical menopause" occurs and hormone replacement therapy is usually considered.

Most women get through the menstrual irregularities of peri-menopause without diagnostic or therapeutic procedures. However, the best "take-home" message of this chapter is to keep a diary/menstrual calendar to keep track of your menses (and to show to your health care provider if necessary). If you have a disturbing pattern or if your heavy menses/bleeding are fatiguing you, your calendar will be of help to you and your physician.

## Types of Abnormal Menses

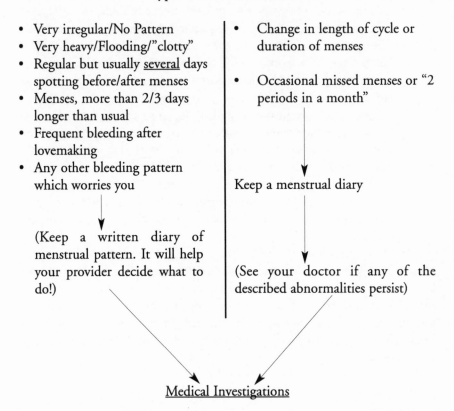

- Very irregular/No Pattern
- Very heavy/Flooding/"clotty"
- Regular but usually <u>several</u> days spotting before/after menses
- Menses, more than 2/3 days longer than usual
- Frequent bleeding after lovemaking
- Any other bleeding pattern which worries you

- Change in length of cycle or duration of menses

- Occasional missed menses or "2 periods in a month"

Keep a menstrual diary

(Keep a written diary of menstrual pattern. It will help your provider decide what to do!)

(See your doctor if any of the described abnormalities persist)

## Medical Investigations

Trial of Hormonal Therapy • Pelvic Ultrasound • Endometrial biopsy • Hysteroscopy • Laparoscopy

## Various Therapeutic Options

(Although it may take a little while to accurately diagnose and treat abnormal uterine bleeding, this should be diagnosed and a viable treatment plan be in place within a maximum of six months...)

## JUDY'S STORY

"I've got my cyst back," Judy announced as I escorted her into my consultation room.

Judy Descartes and I had been through several cysts together. A long-time patient of mine, it was apparently all I could do each time to hold her back from the knife. ("Why don't you just cut it out?" was her usual litany.)

A big woman who knew her own mind, she never hesitated to come in when her cysts were acting up. (She liked seeing the ultrasound pictures of "her insides," as she put it, and the good-natured repartee which had developed between us over the years. She, always asking for me to "cut out" each new and transient cyst (knowing that I wouldn't), and me wondering if she ever was going to let me do something about her periods which, I knew, were getting heavier and heavier. (Her hematocrit, the red blood cell count, was now 33%-normal is 36-44%.) She had been stoically suffering increasingly long and heavy menses for as long as both of us could remember. She was kidding (both of us knew) about removing the cysts. She was definitely afraid of "the knife."

Her pain (this time low on the right side) was back, and in addition to her usual heavy periods (now up to 7-8 days long) she mentioned an unusual episode of spotting beginning 2-3 days before her last period which, she stated, "...lasted forever. I only bled heavy 2-3 days, but then it seemed to go on and off for more than a week longer." As an afterthought she added that she had bled lightly after she had made love with her husband the previous night. "Scared the crap out of him," she told me, "although, if I keep bleeding like I am with my periods, which now seem like forever, I won't have to worry about bleeding after sex—there won't be any sex!"

We did our usual ultrasound, in which we located our usual small benign-appearing ovarian cyst ("Don't worry, it will be gone by next month...two at the latest."). Additionally, however, I noticed that the endometrium, the lining tissue inside Judy's uterus, was distinctly thicker than I had remembered it in the past. Although it appeared quite regular in contour, and was probably within normal limits for the late part of her menstrual cycle, I carefully measured it and made a note to check it again when I reimaged her in 2-3 months to reassure us both that the cyst was on its way out (rather than in).

As it turned out, Judy returned sooner than 2-3 months. Six weeks later she was back, this time in the midst of what she referred to as "an energizer bunny" period. "It keeps going on and on and on." She had again spotted for several days prior to her last period, which had never really ended, but just stretched into her next period, which, of course, had ended the day she made the appointment. She had again, she told me, "bled all over Randy," who had kidded her, saying that he finally got to deflower her, an act he had not been party to originally.

We repeated the ultrasound. As expected, the little cyst was history. Her endometrium, however, despite her 35-40 days of spotting/bleeding, was thick as ever, now measuring 15 mm (it had been 14 mm last time). Although it was still mostly symmetrical, with my vaginal probe I thought I could identify some minute vascular spaces (consistent with an endometrial polyp) within the otherwise homogeneous lining.

"I'd like to look a little closer into your endometrium," I told Judy, and I briefly described the procedure of sonohysterography, whereby a small amount of liquid was placed via a slender catheter within the uterus, the resulting liquid acting as a contrast to the uterine tissue, which had a decidedly different echodensity. (I used lidocaine, a local anesthetic, as my contrast media so that if I saw something as I was doing the procedure, I could biopsy it with minimal discomfort at the same time.) In this way, I could "outline" whatever was enlarged in Judy's uterus and distinguish between a polyp and hyperplasia, or thickened endometrium. The latter could be secondary either to the cyst or to increased estrogen levels in relation to progesterone; I could easily get a sample with an endometrial biopsy and most likely this could be easily and successfully treated with several short courses of progesterone therapy.

We scheduled the sonohysterography for that Friday, but Judy canceled, promising to reschedule. When she did not call a week later, I had my secretary phone her. Judy again postponed scheduling, protesting a "packed schedule..." When she still hadn't phoned after another week, I personally called her, suggesting that we meet briefly at no charge to just "talk things over." I suspected that something more was going on than met the eye. The next day, when Judy was seated across from me in my office, I confronted her with my suspicions: "You're scared to death of this, aren't you? You think it might be cancer."

Judy broke down crying. After she'd composed herself, she let her story come out. Her grandmother, who had practically raised her and to whom Judy had been extremely close, had had "a polyp" when Judy was 8. It was on her vocal chords. "It's nothing, sweetie," Nana had told her. "The doctor said it's certainly benign—I just need a minor operation to remove it."

Nana had not survived the "minor operation." The polyp on her vocal chords proved to be malignant, and in the ensuing radical surgery, a major blood vessel had been inadvertently severed. Nana survived the surgery, but not her protracted recovery and had died in the hospital three weeks later, never regaining consciousness, and never providing "closure" with Judy. It had been an extremely traumatic event in the young girl's life.

"When you said polyp, I quietly freaked," Judy admitted. "I just didn't know how to explain it all to you."

I apologized to Judy for being so cavalier in my approach to the proposed diagnostic and therapeutic procedures, and proceeded to more fully explain what an endometrial polyp was. I honestly and quietly admitted the small but very real malignant potential. We talked about polyps everywhere: what they were, how and why they formed, what they did and didn't do, how likely they were to be malignant. When she left my office late that afternoon, Judy was the "polyp maven of Davis".

To make a potentially very long story short, Judy did have her sonohysterography. It did show an approximately 1 x 1.2 x 3 cm typical, smooth-walled, endometrial polyp. It had none of the visual features of malignancy (I'd show you the Polaroids, but they don't print up very well). Judy did great and even watched the whole thing on the video monitor. ("You can't show these," she joked, "without checking with my agent.")

After the somewhat prolonged diagnostic dance, the therapeutic decision was relatively easy. Yes, she was still bleeding, Judy admitted. Yes, her periods (while not of epic proportions) were still, she euphemistically said, "brisk." (Her red blood cell count was now even lower, down to 30.5%.) "Yes," she grudgingly said, "I guess it's about time to have it out."

I counseled her that at the same time as removal of her polyp, I could do a procedure known as "endometrial ablation," where the lining tissue of the uterine cavity was cauterized or "sealed," making it very difficult for the endometrium to re-form, thus (along with her polyp removal) dramatically lowering the amount she would bleed with each cycle. "In 40-50% of the cases there is no bleeding whatsoever," I told her. "In another 40-50% the periods are quite light to normal. There is an approximately 10-20% failure rate" (periods as heavy as usual by a year after the surgery). "Additionally," I counseled her, "your ability to get pregnant after the procedure will be exceedingly rare, and for all practical purposes, especially at your age (Judy was 46), it's also a sterilization procedure."

She certainly perked up with this news. "It's like killing three birds with one stone," she said. "I'd give you the gold medal for that."

Although she was slightly sobered after I gave her the information for full informed consent, as honestly as possible discussing the known risks of the procedures, she proceeded to schedule and then undergo surgery two weeks later. I don't think she truly let her breath out, however, until I phoned her with the "benign" pathology report three days later.

*They're not hot flashes—they're power surges*
—Anonymous

# CHAPTER FIVE

## THE PERI-MENOPAUSE
### "All Over the Map"

Menopause is a normal, natural event, not a disease! As a woman moves from her reproductive years through the transition of menopause and beyond, however, physical and emotional changes most certainly occur.

Similar to the passage through menarche (the beginning of hormonal cycling), the far side of a woman's reproductive years is not an isolated event, but repeats in a perhaps more extensive fashion the years-long passage through adolescence.

At this point, let's again review some definitions:

<u>Peri-Menopause</u> means literally "around menopause." It is that time before and after the actual event of menopause ("...the last menstrual period...") when a woman knows "something is happening" and that "happening" is still going on.

She knows from changes brought on by shifts in hormonal production that she feels different. More ups and downs, poorer sleep, fatigue, memory difficulties, hot flashes and menstrual cycle changes. If left to themselves ("natural menopause"—see below), these symptoms would in most cases spontaneously resolve in approximately 6 months to 2 years after menopause. Although by definition, this transition ends the first year after menopause (the last menstrual period), it can actually last 4-8 years or more.

<u>Natural Menopause</u> is the spontaneous and permanent ending of menstruation, and is not caused by medical intervention. In the Western world, most women experience natural menopause between the ages of 40 and 58 (the average is approximately 51). Some women go through menopause in their late 20s and 30s ("premature menopause") and a few in their late 50s and 60s ("late menopause").

There is a genetic trend to timing of menopause: women more often than not go through menopause around the same age as their mothers and sisters. Other than genetics, cigarette smoking is the only proven factor affecting menopausal age. (Smokers experience menopause 1-2 years earlier than non-smokers.)

Induced Menopause is immediate menopause in response to an external event brought on by surgical removal of pre-menopausal ovaries, cancer chemotherapy, or pelvic irradiation.

A hysterectomy alone (removal of the uterus only), with ovaries left in place, does not induce menopause. Confusing sometimes is the term "total hysterectomy." Medically, this refers to removal of the entire uterus (with the cervix, the lower part of the uterus), but does not include ovarian removal (this would be a "total hysterectomy with salpingo oophorectomy"). In laymen's terms, however, a "total" or "complete" hysterectomy is used erroneously to describe removal of the uterus and ovaries.

If you have had uterine surgery, or radiation or chemotherapy for cancer, make sure that your doctor puts in writing (for future reference) exactly what was removed and why. Also, be sure to discuss what this means regarding the possible need for immediate and long term hormone replacement therapy.

Although occasionally a simple hysterectomy disturbs blood supply to the ovaries causing hot flashes, women who have had a hysterectomy still go through peri-menopause and menopause as their ovaries secrete less estrogen. It's just that they no longer have the reliable "marker" of their menses and attendant irregularity to help evaluate where they are.

There is no peri-menopause with an induced menopause. Because of the abrupt loss of ovarian hormones, the menopausal disturbance of hot flashes and mood alterations can be much more intense than the gradual adjustment of "natural menopause." Additionally, if prompt hormonal replacement therapy is not undertaken, these women spend more time without the protective effect of estrogen on bone and possibly heart, putting them at greater risk for osteoporosis and possibly heart disease.

Emotionally also, the impact of induced menopause may be greater than with natural menopause, as frequently these women must cope with both the disease or condition which led to their earlier-than-expected menopause and frequently with side effects of adjunctive cancer therapy, in addition to the sudden menopausal symptoms.

It's a tough place to be, and women in this situation experience uncertainty, confronting menopause and balancing the dynamic relationship between menopause and cancer in their lives.

Of importance is this: If you are pre-menopausal and are contemplating surgical removal of ovaries, or if a cancer in your body necessitates therapy by radiation or chemotherapy, make sure, well before these procedures, that you sit down with your doctor and discuss the ramifications of the procedure on your hormones. What will happen here? What are your alternatives? Should you take hormone replacement therapy (HRT)? What about testosterone? What are the ramifications of taking HRT on your primary disease? What are the risks of <u>not</u> taking HRT? Will plant sources and/or non-hormonal therapy help?

Do not have the surgery/therapy until these issues are worked out. The time to do so is <u>before</u> (not after) therapy. Make sure your doctor makes time to discuss this, or refers you to someone who can help you with an intelligent, comfortable decision and treatment plan. (More about this in later chapters...)

<u>Premature Menopause</u> is menopause reached before the age of 40. This occurs in approximately 5% of women. Although most women experiencing premature menopause do so in their 30s, cessation of ovulation is not rare in one's 20s.

Premature menopause may be the result of genetics, an "*autoimmune* process," or medical interventions (see above).

By autoimmune, I mean some alteration in the functioning of the immune system of your body which serves to prematurely inactivate or destroy primordial or pre-developing egg follicles, depleting the ovaries of their egg supply.

Premature menopause places a woman at increased risk for osteoporosis and possibly heart disease over the rest of her life.

Because premature menopause signals the end of natural childbearing, it can cause significant distress for women and couples who have not completed their families. Premature menopause can generate additional significant psychological issues also, as many women link their femininity and sexual desirability with their fertility.

If you experience premature menopause, in addition to discussing the importance of hormone replacement therapy and the options available to you with your health care provider, make sure that you explore your inner feelings and the psychological impact of this change with your practitioner or therapist.

<u>Post-Menopause</u> is all the years after menopause, whether natural or induced.

### How Does One Confirm Menopausal Status?

Hormonal testing is usually not necessary to confirm that a woman has gone through menopause, since therapy, if required, is usually based on a woman's symptoms or concerns. If a woman is in her 40s or 50s and is bothered by the typical symptoms of shifting and lowered hormonal levels (e.g., hot flashes, mood alterations, etc.)...maybe her periods are regular, maybe not—therapy is usually based on symptoms, not on hormone levels.

If you are a doctor, what are you going to do if a woman is significantly symptomatic? Check hormone levels, and if they are not abnormal, say "I'm sorry, dear, your hormone levels are normal; I'm not going to treat you. The symptoms must all be in your head. Just go home and don't worry about it." I should think not!

Hormone levels can be misleading since estrogen production does not steadily fall during menopause, but usually fluctuates with days, weeks, or months of fairly high or low levels. It is these fluctuations rather than actual or average levels which cause the symptoms. It would take months of daily and weekly testing to make sense of it.

That said, there definitely are times when isolated hormone testing makes sense: when it will have some impact on you and your physician's mutual decision whether to or how to treat.

FSH (follicle stimulating hormone) is the hormone put out by the pituitary gland in the brain to regulate the ovaries. If the ovaries are working fine and there is plenty of estrogen, these estrogen levels effectively shut off the pituitary's secretion of FSH, and levels are low. If, however, estrogen levels are chronically low, FSH levels elevate. It's like the pituitary is flogging the ovaries, as if to say, "C'mon, ovaries, do it! do it! Put out more estrogen!" An FSH test, therefore, will be quite elevated, indicating the pituitary gland's response to chronically low estrogen levels.

Where FSH testing can be especially helpful is when, for some reason (e.g., whether or not to operate on symptomatic fibroids) it would be nice to know approximately how close a woman is to her natural menopause. For this, make sure your practitioner orders your FSH for the second or third day of your menstrual cycle, or does what is called a "Clomiphene Challenge Test," where, after the cycle day 2/3 FSH you take the "fertility pill" Clomid® for 5 days, after which the FSH is repeated. This is a good way to approximate ovarian reserve (whether you've got plenty of eggs left or are perhaps "running low" and menopause is imminent).

**Peri-Menopausal Issues:**

    1. Fertility and Contraception

Yes, you can still get pregnant at 50 (although it's not terribly likely. Better stated: It's downright rare). What are your odds? At whatever age in your peri-menopausal years, if you are symptomatic (hot flashes, mood swings, irregular menses) your odds of pregnancy are less than if you have no symptoms and your menses are mostly regular. To give you a very rough idea, the per-cycle odds of a woman in her 20s who makes love every 2-3 days having a positive pregnancy test is ±35-40%. The same scenario at age 40 is ±3-5%, dropping to 1-2% (at best) at age 45. (Of course, if you're making love only once a week or once a month, the odds drop considerably!)

The same contraceptive options (including female and male sterilization) available to younger women can be used by women in their

40s, keeping in mind that oral contraceptives are not a good choice for a woman who smokes, has a strong family history of heart disease at a younger age, or is at high risk for a blood clot in her legs (poor circulation, sedentary lifestyle, deep varicose veins, history of previous blood clot).

In a non-smoking woman without risk factors, especially if she is having irregular menses (with no disease conditions found after a workup) or beginning to suffer from mild peri-menopausal symptoms, birth control pills, patch, or vaginal ring can be a fine option with which to provide both birth control and segue into menopause (switching to standard HRT later if necessary and/or desired).

If diminished sexual desire is part of your equation, however, birth control pills might not be the best option. Birth control pills (and all oral estrogens) elevate a blood protein called "sex hormone binding globulin" (SHBG). SHBG binds free testosterone, taking much of it out of circulation. If your sex drive is already low, this further suppression in addition to already low testosterone levels may be like trading a headache for an upset stomach.

2. Changes in Bleeding Patterns (see Chapter 4)

3. Hot Flashes

Hot flashes (or hot flushes, if you're a poker player) are, along with menstrual irregularities, always a part of peri-menopause. Whether at night (where frequently they are the most noticeable) and/or daytime, whenever they occur they are a bother—anywhere from a nuisance to a major disruption. They are the result of sudden changes in the hypothalamus, the center of the brain that acts as the body's thermostat. This center is acutely sensitive to shifting hormonal levels, and, among other things, responds by "tweaking" the tiny nerves which serve the tiny blood vessels (capillaries) of the skin, causing them to dilate, or open more, producing a feeling of heat on the skin: both "flashing" and "flushing." Sometimes this is so intense that "the sweat just rolls off."

Night sweats obviously interfere with sleep (fluctuating estrogen levels, even without sweats, can disrupt patterns of healthy deep sleep;—remember the REM sleep discussed in the PMS chapter?). This chronically poor sleep causes fatigue, which may lead to irritability.

While for a given woman, hot flashes usually have a consistent pattern, that pattern differs from woman to woman. In some, they are only a minor annoyance, while in others, they can be debilitating. Most peri-menopausal women who experience flashes do so for several years, but some only for a short time. That's part of the hassle: not knowing when they will stop!

Much of the time, if you take a moment to think about it, you can identify particular triggers that seem to bring on the flash, such as heat (hair dryer, warm room, etc.), hot drinks, spicy foods, strong emotions, etc. Some drug therapies prescribed for women for breast cancer chemotherapy (tamoxifen) or HRT/osteoporosis prevention (raloxifen or "Evista®") can cause hot flashes.

<u>So, how can you get rid of them?</u>

There are several methods I recommend as first line therapy. Frequently these provide enough relief to make things tolerable. These include:

\* Exercise regularly! Vigorous exercise releases endorphins, increasing serotonin in the brain, reducing stress and promoting better sleep.

\* Further diminish stress by the use of meditation, yoga, massage, a leisurely bath, etc. (see Chapter 13).

\* Avoid hot flash <u>triggers</u> (listed above).

\* Keep cool! (Lightweight clothing, fan, etc.)

If these measures are insufficient, there are many hormonal (next chapter), herbal, botanical, and non-hormonal (Chapter 7) therapies that you can rely on.

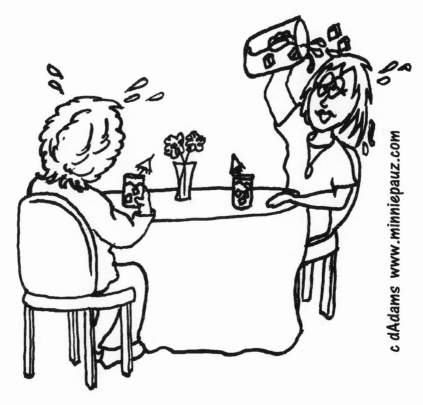

# Hot Flash Treatment #10...A pitcher of iced tea

4. Sleep Difficulties

Similar to PMS sufferers, insomnia appears to be very common in the peri-menopause. Whether it is from hot flashes/night sweats (It's hard to get quality REMs when you're drenched with perspiration!) or from stress secondary to other disturbances of the menopause (it's definitely a "chicken and egg" phenomenon), sleep quality is frequently poor in the peri-menopause.

What helps? Well, getting the sweats under control certainly goes a long way! (See above and Chapters 6 and 7). Lifestyle changes including daily exercise (but not near bedtime), avoiding coffee, alcohol and nicotine, and avoiding heavy meals in the evening help. Adjusting the levels of ambient light, noise and temperature as well as a "bedtime ritual" (Chapter 13) also help ease insomnia.

5. Sexuality/Sexual Function Changes

Sexual concerns are common in midlife women and are discussed in much greater detail in Chapter 8.

For present purposes, suffice it to say that a general decrease in sexual desire is almost the norm in midlife women. Whether it is secondary to hormonal issues (especially decreasing testosterone levels from the ovaries), peri-menopausal issues such as fatigue, depression, and a general feeling of "lack of sexiness" resulting from fluctuating estrogen levels or partnership issues (marital stress, "sameness") or a little of both, is hard to say. It's probably a combination of all of these things but, as you will see in Chapter 8, there are definitely ways of determining what is the cause and working with this to successfully regain an enjoyable sexual life. (Of course, if your sex life is fine or if diminished sexual desire is not an issue in your life at this time, there's no reason to do anything about it. "If it ain't broke, don't fix it!")

6. Fatigue and Psychological Changes

If you are up half the night with hot flashes (and disturbed about them during the daytime), experiencing mood swings that you do not have control of, are late for work the second time this week because you've forgotten where you put your keys, and are worried about the cause of your irregular bleeding pattern...of course you'd be fatigued!

During reproductive years, most women become accustomed to their individual hormonal rhythms. But during peri-menopause the rhythm changes. (Try dancing to Disco when R&B is in your soul.) These fluctuations, while "normal" can sure contribute to mood swings.

Or not! EVERY WOMAN IS INDIVIDUAL, and each experiences her passage into midlife in her own individual way.

The idea is to create or maintain balance in your own personal life, to balance the obligations of work and caring for others with the self-nurturing that is even more important in these years. There are many potential sources of stress during midlife, including relationship problems, divorce or widowhood, care for children (especially struggles with adolescents), being childless, frequently not by choice (see Chapter 18), concerns and caregiving responsibilities for aging parents, changing career issues, and body changes associated with aging. In our youth-oriented society, getting older can be especially difficult, and midlife women often see changes in self-esteem, self-concept, and body image.

Just <u>recognizing</u> these problematic issues can lead to better understanding and the desire to learn the coping skills to empower you to meet these challenges, renew self confidence, and restore balance and harmony (see especially Chapter 13).

If your coping skills aren't sufficient to relieve the symptoms of stress, it's a good idea to see a health care practitioner you trust. Your feelings may be a side effect of medication you are taking, or may be the result of depression for which therapy and/or medication might be very helpful.

General irritability and "blue moods" can often be relieved by lifestyle changes (e.g., exercise) and working on the <u>balances</u> just discussed. Relaxation, stress reduction techniques, and frequently hormone replacement therapy can help many women cope with life's stress factors during this time of hormonal fluctuation. Mood disturbances brought on by sleep deprivation resulting from hot flashes usually improve when hot flashes are treated.

If you're still depressed, though (symptoms of persistent fatigue, disinterest in friends, job, sex; seemingly uncontrollable mood swings, etc.), medication may be needed.

You might first try an herbal remedy such as St. John's Wort (300 mg 3 times a day), while at the same time seeking "talk therapy" with a professional such as a marriage and family counselor (MFC), licensed clinical social worker (LCSW), clinical psychologist (PhD), psychiatrist (MD), minister, or even a perceptive friend or neighbor.

Clinical depression is not specifically related to menopause, but is associated with a chemical imbalance in the brain. If clinical depression is found to be contributing to your symptoms, one of a variety of very effective prescription antidepressant medications can be prescribed to successfully correct this imbalance (but remember: antidepressant medication is best used in combination with counseling and psychotherapy).

Anxiety (a heightened sense of anticipation, dread or fear), although experienced by most everyone at one time or another, may be more common in peri-menopausal women. If it tends to be persistent, the herb Kava-Kava

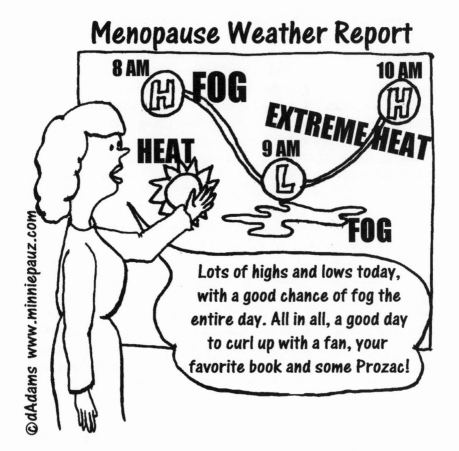

(see Chapter 7) and/or conscious breath medication (slow conscious in-and-out breathing (see Chapter 13) help significantly. If anxiety occurs with other symptoms of peri-menopause, HRT (Reminder: this stands for hormone replacement therapy) may be helpful. For occasional relief from severe anxiety, the medication Xanax® may be helpful. Panic disorder, a psychological condition resulting in recurrent shortness of breath, chest pain, dizziness, heart palpitations and/or feelings of "going crazy," warrants psychotherapy and/or medical combinations. Sometimes, also, anxiety symptoms can be related to depression.

Peri-menopausal women frequently report difficulty concentrating and minor memory problems. You are probably not losing your mind, nor do you have Alzheimer's (despite what your teenagers may say)! While these problems may be as related to stress as they are to the hormonal shifts of the peri-menopause, estrogen frequently provides relief, as do some herbal remedies (e.g., Estrovan® or Remifemin® or other combinations including black cohosh)—but less reliably.

Although so often people are reluctant to seek the services of a psychiatrist or therapist, no one should suffer in silence. Tell someone if these things are going on and not being relieved. Your family doc or ob-gyn should be able to recommend someone (or help herself/himself). Ask your friends regarding a good therapist. Frequently your clergyperson (Is that politically correct?) can help.

7. Urogenital Changes

Many women notice midlife changes involving their vulva, vagina, and bladder functions.

They find themselves drier during lovemaking, producing less lubrication and with occasional irritation. They are more prone to vulvar burning, itching, or pain. They frequently notice urinary urgency: a very pressing need to urinate RIGHT NOW, and more frequently leak urine when coughing or exercising.

Sexual relations can become more uncomfortable with this loss of lubrication, leading to less enjoyment, difficulty in achieving orgasm, and withdrawal from lovemaking. Lubrication is hugely helpful here (and will be discussed in greater detail in Chapter 8). A "personal lubricant" such as Astroglide®, Lubrin®, etc., or a light oil (baby oil, massage oil, light olive oil, etc.) rubbed between the hands to warm and applied lovingly, sparingly, or lavishly to appropriate anatomical areas can be lots of fun while providing good lubrication as well.

These changes range from only mildly annoying to debilitating. Their causes vary and so does the treatment (see Chapters 6, 8, and 15).

Vulvo-vaginal changes occur as a result of natural decreases in estrogen levels, causing tissues of the vulva and vagina to atrophy (become thin, dryer and less elastic); pubic hair can wane (women's answer to male pattern baldness?) and, especially with lack of regular sexual stimulation and adequate estrogen levels, the vaginal wall can become shorter and narrower and more prone to minor fissures and tears, especially during lovemaking. Prescription estrogen therapy (oral, transdermal, or locally applied vaginal) usually rapidly restores thickness and elasticity of these tissues. (See next chapter.) A diet high in soy foods or soy supplements helps some women, although it may take months to see results.

The diminished estrogen levels of approaching menopause may cause the lining of the urethra to become thin and the surrounding muscles may weaken. This may lead to a greater incidents of urinary frequency, urgency ("...gotta go, gotta go"), nocturia (getting up a lot at night to pee), stress incontinence (using urine when you cough, laugh, lift, sneeze, etc.), and dysuria (hurts when you go). This is all discussed in detail (including therapies) in Chapter 15.

8. <u>Other Health Changes</u>

No, you're not falling apart (it just seems that way!), but make no mistake about it, your body <u>is</u> changing:

* It's easier to gain weight (And harder to lose it!)
* Heart palpitations (Caused by fluctuating hormone levels? Anxiety? Thyroid disease, though this is unlikely?) are more common.
* It's stiffer getting out of bed in the morning.
* Headaches (Tension? Migraine?) are more common.
* Loss of collagen and elasticity causes wrinkles and sags (especially in long-time smokers)
* Your hair is gray (at least at the roots) and may be thinning to boot.
* Eyes...?? Teeth...??

OK, OK! It's natural to age. But you sure can do it more evenly, gracefully; more happily. How?? Basic Stuff:

1. Don't smoke! In every which way, smoking gets you. (Early menopause, more hot flashes, poor skin tone, chronic and sometimes fatal lung and heart problems, increased rate of colon cancer, etc., etc.) How to quit: Hypnosis classes, gum, patches, antidepressants, "cold turkey." You have to replace it with <u>something</u>. (How about #2, below?)

2. EXERCISE. If I had to name one panacea or "cure-all," it would be exercise. Fast walking (especially while swinging light weights), running, biking, swimming, aerobics, weights and machines, ball playing, tennis, etc. The important thing is to be sweating and perhaps a little out of breath.

An important point: <u>Do not look on exercise as fun!</u> Sure, certain exercises (e.g., tennis and frequent social aspects of fast walking with friends, etc.) may be pleasant, but usually <u>exercise is work</u>. But, unequivocally, necessary, important work.

Less hot flashes, less cancer and heart disease, better skin tone, less depression and better mood. You name it, exercise makes it better.

Insofar as weight loss goes, unfortunately there's <u>no free lunch</u>. For every 10 pounds that have been lost with Metabolife® or whatever pill, potion or magic diet you care to name, <u>13 lbs.</u> have been gained!

Whatever your temporary or permanent physical limitation, <u>there is an exercise for you!</u>

3. Better diet and vitamins. "You are what you eat." It's true. I don't make many "all or none" didactic statements in this book, but when it comes to exercise and proper nutrition, I sure do. There is nothing to substitute for eating the right amount of the right kind of foods.

What's good: Fresh fruits and veggies, grains (cornmeal, rice, wheat, pasta). Beans and peas: lentils, garbanzos, limas, pintos, snap beans, etc., etc.

Fish. Some chicken (cook it with the skin on and then take most of the skin off before eating). Occasional meat (go low on the fatty stuff).

Death? Deep fried, fatty, "smothered," "oozing," "piled high," "buttery," "supersized"... you get the picture.

There is no way to alter your diet away from the greasy and toward the fresh-n-natural without getting your family involved. If you've all been brought up on fast foods and lots of meat-n-potatoes, just try serving them stir-fried veggies and tofu and see what happens! But how about a huge salad with chunks of tuna, cubes of ham or chicken, garbanzos, kidney beans, slices of tofu, nuts, peppers, olives, shrimp, imitation crab meat, veggies, etc., etc., along with a good hunk of French bread dipped in flavored olive oil. Or a bowl of pasta with marinara sauce and olives, mushrooms, light sausage or clams, seafood, etc.; or lean chicken, veggies, etc. Or stir fry of veggies and strips of lean meat served over rice. Or polenta with tomato sauce and lean meat on top. Or couscous with lemon chicken and raisins.

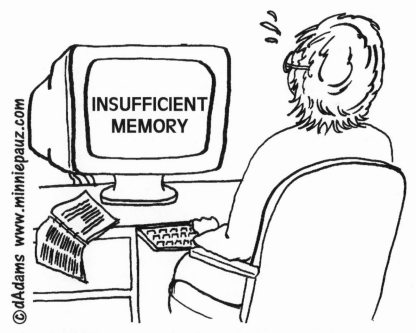

**Oh great, now my computer is having menopausal symptoms!**

Bean casseroles. Steamed veggies. Fruit salads. Etc., etc. You'll <u>feel better</u>. You'll <u>feel stronger</u>. You'll <u>look better</u>. You'll <u>be healthier</u> and less likely to croak at 59 from a coronary or stroke (much less cancer too).

Vitamins? A good balanced mega B, 500-1000 mg vitamin C, 400 I.U. vitamin E, 800 I.U. vitamin D, 1000-1500 mg calcium and 500-1000 mg magnesium. Others you can add in depending on your desires and orientation.

So, there it is. It is what it is. And the chapters ahead will help you deal with it all!

## WINN'S STORY

The first thing out of Winn's mouth, even before she was seated in my consultation room at her first visit, was that she "didn't like doctors." Something about my ad in a local newspaper had caught her eye (or rather her partner's eye) and she thought she'd "Give it a shot."

A truck driver, Winn looked to be in her mid-40s (she was 44), maybe 60-80 lbs. overweight, dressed in loose jeans and a sweatshirt. She had one grown daughter and was in a relatively new relationship with a woman who was the dispatcher at one of the trucking companies she drove for.

"It was Bonnie who got me to come, actually," Winn admitted. "We get along real well, but lately I've been, well, sorta biting her head off..." Winn had not had good prior experiences with the "medical establishment." In her mid 30s, a period of real upheaval in her life, she was briefly institutionalized for "depression" and medicated ("gorked out") by medical staff who "...took all my decisions away from me. I had no choice," she lamented when I asked her about why she was so down on doctors and their therapies. "There was no listening or explaining involved; I was just given drugs."

Eventually she recovered, radically changing professions (and preferred sexual orientation) and was doing generally well "...until my periods started going wacko and my mood started yo-yoing." She had (reluctantly) gone to her HMO doctor, who had ordered an FSH, found it to be "normal," and sent Winn on her way saying, "Well, the test shows you're not in menopause. Come back in 6 months if it's still a problem." He'd offered her birth control pills to "regulate the periods," but without need for contraception, a general distrust of medication and the fact that she still smoked cigarettes occasionally, Winn had declined.

As is my habit at initial consultations, I explained that we had all the time we needed to make sure that we got all of her issues "on the table," and then to prioritize and combine, as indicated. "You might be here 'til midnight." she quipped.

First and foremost were the mood changes. "I thought it was PMS at first and, yes it is worse before my periods (though I never can figure out when one is coming). But it's really all the time now and I don't like it!"

As we got onto other things, she related some nighttime hot flashes, but not much of a bother. She certainly wasn't sleeping well, but was unsure whether to pin that on the flashes, getting up 3-4 times to pee, or waking up at 4 a.m., unable to fall back to sleep.

"...and my libido's in the toilet," she added, almost as an afterthought, although I could see by the worried and frustrated look on her face that this was a bigger deal than she let on.

"Bonnie 'n me had a real good sex life at first, but now I guess I could care less if I get any or not. Bonnie's getting tired of having to ask all the time."

As we got into the matter in more detail, I was to find that her periods also weren't as regular as they had been. "It's not like I really <u>miss</u> any," Winn said, "but I'm never quite sure when one'll come. I used to be regular 28 days. Now they're mostly every 3-3½ weeks, but sometimes I wait almost a month and a half..."

"My memory was never that great," she admitted, "but it's definitely worse now, and I'm more moody. Although it's all worse before my periods, it's not just then that I notice it."

Continuing the process of "discovery," we went on to talk about some minor problems with urinary urgency (a couple of times recently she'd wet her pants on the way to the bathroom) and her having to get up several times at night to pee.

We then went on to her eating habits and day-by-day activities. "I mostly eat on the run. That or truck stop food," she said. I scanned the "food diary" for the past 24 hours that she'd filled out on her intake form. "<u>Breakfast</u>: Egg McMuffin and coffee. <u>Lunch</u>: Hamburger, fries and a coke ('ketchup for my vegetable,' she had added). <u>Supper</u>: Tuna casserole with cheese and chips on top. <u>Snacks</u>: Bag of chips; coffee; an apple." (I told her I liked the apple!)

Under "Exercise" on the form she had listed "none."

Her physical exam was essentially unremarkable except for a borderline elevated blood pressure (140/90) and the fact that she was more than a little overweight. Pelvic exam was fine and I took a Pap smear.

We discussed the concept of peri-menopause and I gave her the North American Menopause Society's "Menopause Guidebook" to peruse before her next visit. We arranged for a mammogram (Her last one was 5 years before!), a colonoscopy (both her father and an older brother had had colon cancer; her brother at age 51), and some lab work: a lipid profile, homocysteine, c-Reactive Protein, TSH (to check thyroid status), and salivary testosterone (to roughly evaluate tissue levels of testosterone). She asked about "...a test to see when I'm going through menopause," and I replied that unfortunately there was no such animal. "I might find that it looks like you're nearing menopause, and I might not," I explained. "The test is not terribly accurate. The treatment is really based on your symptoms, not on lab values which tend to shift often in the peri-menopause."

Winn returned a week later. Her mammography and colonoscopy hadn't been done yet, but her other lab had, and she'd read most of the Menopause Guidebook.

"Your thyroid's fine," I said (her test result was in the normal range) "Your salivary testosterone is a tad low; we'll talk more about that later. But I'm worried about your lipids."

Winn's total cholesterol was modestly elevated, but her other blood lipids, coupled with slightly elevated triglycerides were disturbing. LDL (the bad cholesterol) and VLDL (the very bad cholesterol) both were modestly elevated, and the HDLs (high density lipoproteins, or the "good" or protective cholesterol) was low. "Some of this could be familial or genetic," I told her. "But I'll bet most of it is caused by your lifestyle. Your diet sure promotes the elevated LDLs and your lack of exercise and perhaps relatively low estrogen levels lead to the poor (low) HDLs. In fact, her "bad" to "good" cholesterol ratios and coronary risk status were both elevated into the danger zone.

"Well, son of a gun," Winn grumbled. "All I was interested in when I came here was getting my mood better and my sex drive back—maybe with a couple of hormones—and now you got me scared I might croak." Her tone was chiding, but not angry.

"Oh, I'm keeping your desires in plain view," I told her. "It's just that we might get there in a little of a round-about way. It would be a shame to have you stroking out when you become orgasmic again."

We started discussing ways that, given Winn's work routine, she could improve her dietary habits, adding grains, complex carbohydrates, fresh fruit and vegetables. I advised having fresh fruits, dried fruits, carrots and celery and cereal bars in the cab of her truck for snacks, and drinking lots of water. Shopping for lunch at the salad/deli counter of a supermarket rather than a fast food outlet. Using olive oil instead of butter, cutting down on fat, meats, and deep fried and substituting pasta, stir-frieds, big salads, etc. "You are what you eat," I told her (she groaned). "An adage old but true."

And exercise! "The best way to get your HDLs up. And you'd be surprised at the effects it will have on your mood, your sleep habits, and even your sex drive." We fashioned a routine where she would carry 5 and 10 lb. barbells in a box in her sleeper cab which she would use for 15-20 minutes every morning after arising. And when she took a driving break (or at a truck stop), she'd get in at least 20-30 minutes of fast walking, swinging 2 lb. weights. There was a 24-hour fitness center not far from her home (her girlfriend was already a member) and we worked out an exercise routine for the days she wasn't on the road.

We made a plan to repeat the lipids tests in 3-4 months. I wouldn't hesitate to prescribe a statin, an excellent lipid-lowering medication, I told her, if the lipids were still off kilter.

Winn was going to be on the road for 2 weeks, but we scheduled an appointment for when she returned. I invited her to bring Bonnie along..

When Winn returned, she made sure I knew her muscles were "very sore." "Proves I've been doing my exercises," she grumbled. She was even sleeping better, she grudgingly admitted. Along with the exercise program, Winn had cut down on tobacco and was now smoking "only 2-3 cigarettes a day." We spent the session discussing the pros and cons of very low dose estrogen replacement therapy (either oral or transdermal, but I recommended transdermal in view of the lowered libido and salivary testosterone), to "smooth out the peaks and the valleys," vs. trying herbal products such as Estrovan® (containing red clover and black cohosh) or Promensil® (red clover) plus Remifemin® (an old time and popular black cohosh preparation). "Both of these will probably help with your mood and memory symptoms and the mild hot flashes," I said, "although the estrogens are probably somewhat more reliable and will take less time." We talked about the pros and cons of birth control pills in helping with cycle regulation. We both decided against them. The estrogens, I told her, might also help her urinary urgency and getting up several times at night to void. If she didn't take them, she might try an estrogen vaginal cream to "estrogenize the base of the bladder." She might also get benefit from one of a couple of "bladder relaxant medications," and we made plans for a therapeutic trial.

I offered Winn the option of a trial of transdermal testosterone gel or lotion, along with a couple of counseling sessions with her and Bonnie, discussing sensate focusing (where attention is deliberately and methodically focused on bodily sensations), giving new ideas, specific sensate suggestions and permission to use them. I gave Winn my handout on "Stress Reduction" and meditation techniques and scheduled an appointment to discuss this and a "bedtime ritual" (see Chapter 13), to be modified to fit her trucker's schedule. "Get you sleeping better and we are halfway there," I told her.

We had a long way to go, I knew. But it was a start. What had seemed like a quagmire when she came in was coming into focus, and some resolution was in sight.

Winn's story is...a work in progress.

*The majority of people live below the level of belief or doubt. It takes application and a kind of genius to believe anything, and to believe anything...will probably become more and more difficult as time goes on.*

—T.S. Eliot, *The Enemy*

# CHAPTER SIX

## TO HORMONE OR NOT TO HORMONE
### (...That Is the Question)

This is a story where everyone wins. It is <u>your</u> story, and <u>you</u> get to write the epilogue.

As you read this, neither of us knows exactly what the latest regulations regarding hormone replacement will be by chapter's end. In both medical and lay press, confounding and conflicting studies and recommendations abound.

This chapter will unravel the mystery. Should I take? Why? Should I not take? Why? Herbs? Synthetics? Bioidenticals? (Bioidenticals are hormones synthesized from plant sources to duplicate hormones in the body.) Pills? Patches? Creams, lotions or other potions?

Hormones. Hormones! Nature's panacea or industry's synthetic time bomb? (Neither, actually...) By chapter's end, you will be state-of-the-art educated (and probably more up-to-date than many of the physicians in your community!).

(<u>Please note</u>: In discussing hormone therapy, we will be covering mostly synthetic and bioidentical substances. Although we will also be covering herbs and botanicals, the major evaluation of these will occur in the next chapter.)

### DEFINITIONS
So that we all know what we're talking about here, let me start with a few brief basic definitions (not every topic/concept is being defined here, only the ones that may be a bit confusing to the reader).

1. <u>Estrogen; an estrogen.</u>

Estrogen is a substance produced mainly in the ovary by the cells surrounding the developing egg follicles. Its production is cyclic, rhythmic, and starts at menarche and ends at menopause. Estrogens and compounds that the body metabolizes into estrogens are to a lesser extent produced at other sites in the body (e.g., the adrenal glands, and by fat cells). The three basic types of estrogens are estradiol, estriol and estrone (the latter produced in both the ovary and adrenals; the former two mostly in the ovaries). By metabolic action of the body, however, estrogens are broken down into substances similar to those produced by the breakdown of fat in the body. Even testosterone (also produced by the ovary) follows similar metabolic pathways.

Synthetic or naturally produced by the body, it all ends up more or less the same. The sometimes considerable differences are the "stops along the way." Although estrogens affect mood regulation, emotions, bone density, cardiac health, skin and bone health and temperature regulation, their main activity is to begin to build up a lining in the uterus in preparation for pregnancy implantation and to help nurture that pregnancy along the way. (translation: "preservation of the species...").

If one were to devise a "strength comparison chart," the strongest estrogen by far is the "natural product," put out by a woman's own ovaries. A distant second are the estrogens in oral contraceptives. Third in comparative strength are the estrogens commonly used for hormone replacement therapy, and way back in last place, strengthwise, would be botanicals and phytoestrogens. (Phytoestrogens are plant compounds that have estrogen-like effects in the body.)

2.  Progesterone, "The other female hormone"

Progesterone is produced cyclicly by a woman's ovaries after ovulation (no ovulation, no progesterone).

This substance, produced by the corpus luteum (the area of the ovary where ovulation just took place), serves to "mature" the lining within the uterus built up in response to estrogen stimulation, and to get it ready for implantation of a fertilized egg. If implantation takes place, progesterone continues to be produced by the ovary's corpus luteum until the pregnancy is advanced enough to "stand on its own" (2-3 months). Progesterone is a bit thermogenic—it causes a slight temperature rise in the body. That's why your temperature goes up a few tenths of a degree after ovulation and progesterone production.

If pregnancy and implantation does not occur by a week after ovulation, the progesterone production begins to go down and, in 12-14 days after ovulation, a period ensues.

3.  Progestin

A progestin is a synthetic substance designed to mimic the action of progesterone; that is, to "mature" any uterine tissue "built up" by estrogen (e.g., with birth control pills, post-menopausal estrogen supplementation or excess tissue formed in the uterus when a woman doesn't ovulate) and, with its withdrawal, help "produce" a menses. Giving a progestin (or progesterone, for that matter) continuously with or without estrogen, will at first build up tissue, but then after awhile that tissue will thin and atrophy. Frequently, there is irregular bleeding while this process is occurring.

4.   SERMs (or "Selective Estrogen Receptor Modulators")

Get used to this name; SERMs may be the future of peri- and post-menopausal therapy. Not an estrogen, a Selective Estrogen Receptor Modulator is a synthesized compound that "mimics" an estrogen to the degree that it fills estrogen receptor sites in peripheral tissues. The estrogen receptor (the responsive areas in women's tissue) is very promiscuous; it will "accept" almost anything that looks like an estrogen, even a synthetic with a slightly different configuration. This is how SERMs can produce estrogen-like effects in some tissues and block the estrogen receptor in others, leading to an effect opposite to that of estrogen. It fools the body into thinking that it's an estrogen, but doesn't have estrogen's possible negative side effects on the breasts and uterine lining (endometrium). In fact, presently available SERMs lessen significantly the risk of getting breast cancer. SERMs act to decrease bone turnover and low density lipoprotein cholesterol (the "bad cholesterol").

The problem with presently available SERMs is that they have no beneficial effect whatsoever on the menopausal symptoms of hot flashes, mood and memory changes, etc. (In fact, they may make these worse.)

The present (first generation) SERMs include raloxifene (trade name Evista®), but newer SERMs in research stages or already being used in other countries provide bone density and cardioprotective effects while at the same time mitigating the disturbing menopausal side effects for which most women start HRT in the first place.

Even though SERMs are not estrogens (although they have been erroneously called "designer estrogens"), they in a way fall under the umbrella and may be included under the heading of "hormone replacement therapy."

5.   Oral contraceptive pills (OCPs or BCPs)

Birth control pills are a combination of synthetic estrogens and progestins utilized for cycle regulation and contraception while providing a relatively constant level of hormone replacement. As such, OCPs are frequently utilized in peri-menopausal women who have irregular cycles and other disturbing peri-menopausal symptoms, while at the same time providing contraception, if needed. They can be an excellent transition between peri-menopausal cycle regulation and ongoing lower dose estrogen supplementation therapy.

# COFFEE SHOP

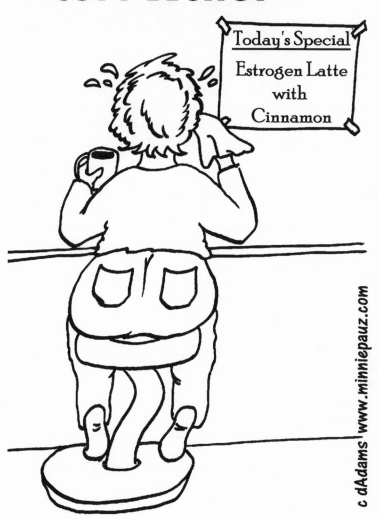

Today's Special

Estrogen Latte
with
Cinnamon

c dAdams www.minniepauz.com

6.  HRT vs. ERT

"HRT" means "hormone replacement therapy" and refers to the administration of <u>both</u> an estrogen <u>and</u> progesterone, or a progestin, either sequentially or in combination. "ERT" means "estrogen replacement therapy" and refers to the administration of an estrogen alone for hormonal replacement.

However, the term "replacement" is a misnomer because ERT/HRT provides only a small fraction of the estrogen once produced by the ovaries. The term "estrogen supplementation" would be much more accurate.

The administration of testosterone is a separate issue, and may be included with either HRT or ERT.

7.  Synthetic

A compound prepared in the laboratory to mimic a naturally occurring substance, or to produce a desired medicinal effect. Examples are the estrogens conjugated estrogen (Premarin®), ethinyl estradiol (the estrogen used in birth control pills), and the progestins medroxyprogesterone acetate (Provera®), norethindrone, and levonorgestrel (the last two also used in birth control pills).

8.  Bioidentical

Also compounded in the laboratory from natural products (such as soybeans or wild Mexican yam) to be "identical" (or nearly so) to naturally occurring substances. Examples include estradiol, estriol, micronized progesterone, and testosterone (in oral or transdermal preparations).

9.  Transdermal

A method of administering hormones so that entry into the body is via absorption through the skin directly into the blood stream (bypassing the GI tract and liver). Transdermals can include matrix patches, where the active substance (e.g. hormone) is imbedded in the plastic polymer and is slowly and constantly absorbed from the polymer for a fixed (4-7 days) period of time (or, in the case of the Estring, a vaginally applied, estrogen-releasing, small diaphragm-like ring, 3 months).

Estradiol as well as testosterone, progesterone, other estrogens and other compounds can also be administered via lozenges or via creams, lotions or gels applied to soft skin (inner arms, inner thighs) for easy absorption.

## WHY TAKE HORMONE THERAPY: WHAT DOES IT DO? WHAT ARE THE RISKS?

If you are taking HRT, you need to ask yourself: "why?" If you are not, you should ask: "why not?"

More than 75% of North American women progressing through peri-menopause and menopause experience hot flashes, as well as associated disturbances such as insomnia and irritability.

If I were writing this chapter a year or two ago, my conclusions and advice would be radically different than they are today. A definite image is beginning to form from all the disparate pieces of observational and evidence-based studies of hormone replacement therapy (Observational = how people appear to do—their feelings about their therapy; evidence-based

= the statistics, the hard, cold facts. Often these two methods produce different results).

"Just <u>why</u> would someone consider taking HRT or ERT?" Well, obviously to replace what's been lost or to help regulate what's there but has become so erratic that your system has all the stability of a bungee jumper off the Golden Gate bridge.

## THE CASE FOR HORMONE REPLACEMENT THERAPY

"...If God had meant for us to have hormones forever, we'd have been born with a heck of a lot more eggs in our ovaries."

I.  The "Medical Reasons"
    1.  <u>Bones</u>: The bone matrix, that which provides the strength, is dynamic. Always breaking down, always being reformed. As long as estrogen is present in a woman and she has enough calcium and performs some amount of weight-bearing exercise, her bone strength will be relatively stable and she won't get osteoporosis. However, after menopause (and in many women during peri-menopause), estrogen levels are not adequate to prevent excessive catabolism (or breakdown) and the bones suffer. Estrogen helps prevent this excessive breakdown (however, other compounds, including testosterone, SERMs, non-hormonal substances such as "bisphosphonates" (Fosamax® or Actonel®) and possibly even the lipid-lowering drugs, the "statins," do the same thing. (See Chapter 9 for more details)
    2.  <u>The Heart</u>: If you don't already have significant heart/vascular disease or hypertension (high blood pressure), estrogen, by means of increasing HDLs (the "good" cholesterol) and decreasing LDLs (the "bad" cholesterol) decreases the risk of coronary vascular disease ("heart disease") and hypertension as you age. However, if you take a progestin (especially medroxyprogesterone acetate or "Provera®"), this beneficial effect is sometimes tempered (natural progesterone has less of a neutralizing action on the positive effects of estrogens).
    3.  <u>Alzheimer's Disease</u>: Depends on who you read... If you have a family history of Alzheimer's, taking low dose estrogens after menopause may statistically lessen your risk of being seriously disabled by this disease. Estrogens are more likely to help if started early (per-menopause) and continued for 10 years or more (low-dose); less likely to help if started late (over age 60). The jury is still out on this one.

4.  Skin tone, hair texture, sense of well being: How much here is placebo effect and how much is directly related to estrogen supplementation is unsure, but women on estrogens generally note a positive effect on their integument (skin and hair) and a general sense of "well being."

5.  Vaginal and urethral health: The so-called "sex skin" (vaginal mucosa) is intrinsically responsive to estrogen levels. Vaginal dryness, burning and trauma during love-making secondary to dryness and thin mucosal skin are all signs of diminishing estrogen levels and can all be controlled by estrogen supplementation, whether oral, transdermal, or direct-vaginal tablet, cream or ring dosing.

6.  Depression: This is new; cutting edge. Although classically depression is managed with counseling and behavioral therapy and/or with medications (classical antidepressants such as the SSRIs (Zoloft®, Prozac®, Paxil®, etc.), anti-epileptics (Klonopin® and Neurontin®), or other medications such as Effexor®, Elavil®, Wellbutrin®, and even St. John's Wort, there is also a hormonal theory of depression. There is a school of thought that in a perhaps sizable minority of women, severe clinical depressive symptoms may be hormonally mediated, from sub-optimal estrogen levels to estrogen excess, requiring natural progesterone (via transdermal cream usually) to mitigate.

    An additional theory holds that estrogen supplementation during peri-menopause (and for some reason not as much after menopause) can help with depressive symptoms.

    If you are suffering from depression and are not doing well on medications or combinations, you may ask your therapist about this. A trial of low dose transdermal estrogen supplementation and/or natural progesterone cream may help where others have failed.

7.  Hearing: Recent studies suggest that a lower level of blood estrogen impedes hearing sensitivity in post-menopausal women.

II. The "Symptomatic Reasons"

Hot flashes. Mood swings. Memory glitches (the so-called "senior moments"). The poor sleep quality, edginess, depression, fatigue. These are all classic peri-menopausal "hormonal swing maladies" (Certainly not melodies!) experienced by a majority of women progressing through menopause that are usually promptly corrected by ERT or HRT.

Yes, after awhile the body gets used to the different hormonal levels and these symptoms frequently diminish on their own. But that "while" might be several years: an uncomfortable length of time to be handicapped. And yes, these symptoms are frequently lessened by botanicals and phyto-estrogens in many women (see Chapter 7), but they take longer to be effective and are less than ideal in probably 50% of women.

With all the questions regarding the true medical indications for HRT/ERT (including the fact that there are non-hormonal agents that may be just as good for these situations), it is the disturbing and frequently debilitating symptoms of peri- and early menopause that lead most women to consider therapy.

And this is probably a very valid and a most reasonable rationale for hormone therapy: to promptly (and safely) manage the difficult twists and changes occurring as one's ovaries begin their swansong.

There is <u>absolutely no evidence</u> that short-term estrogen supple-mentation (defined as under 2-3 and probably for 4-5 years) increases in any way a woman's likelihood of succumbing to breast cancer. A recent meta-analysis ("grand analysis") of more than 45 studies on more than 750,000 women shows no increase in death from breast cancer in women taking short-term (less than 5 years) HRT. Likewise, although previously suspected otherwise, there is no convincing evidence of increased breast cancer rate in women who took birth control pills for many years for either contraceptive or cycle regulation purposes.

## THE CASE AGAINST HRT

Why take something you really do not need? Certainly bone density can be maintained by non-hormonal substances (see Chapter 9). The case for estrogen as a cardiac and vascular system protector (via favorable alterations in blood lipids) is only modestly made, and equally favorable lipid levels can be obtained with a relatively benign class of medications known as "statins" (Zocor®, Lipitor®, Mevacor®...). (See Chapter 11.)

Additionally, although it is acknowledged that estrogens are cardiac and vascular-protective, the risk of an "adverse event" (e.g., heart attack, stroke, blood clot, etc.) taking place is actually higher in the first couple of years after starting HRT <u>in people with a pre-existing history of cardiac or vascular system disease</u> and the risk of thromboembolism (bad blood clot) and gall stones is certainly increased in some women taking hormones. As for the disturbing symptoms of the peri-menopause, significant symptomatic relief can be obtained via botanicals and other non-hormonal agents. (And anyway, these symptoms will usually eventually subside on their own after a period of time.)

Additionally, there are several potential side effects of HRT:

Unscheduled uterine bleeding (starting or returning)

Breast tenderness and occasional enlargement

Abdominal bloating

Fluid Retention

Occasional change in shape of the cornea of the eye, sometimes leading
    to contact lens intolerance

Headaches

Dizziness

Increased breast density, making interpretation of mammograms more
    difficult

Most of these nuisances, however, diminish over time and the majority of women on hormonal supplementation are not significantly affected. All of these potentially adverse effects, especially vaginal bleeding, are minimized by decreasing the dose.

Estrogen does not cause weight gain, but can cause fluid-retention in hands/feet and/or abdominal bloating, sometimes resulting in temporary weight gain.

## WHAT ABOUT PROGESTERONE?

Natural progesterone or a progestin (synthetic), medroxyprogesterone acetate (Provera®) or norethindrone ("NET," Aygestin®). Care usually given either along with estrogen or on a cyclic basis to prevent excessive tissue buildup within the uterus that, in genetically sensitive predisposed individuals, could lead to uterine cancer. However, with ultra-low estrogen dosing (e.g., 0.025 mg patch; 0.3 mg of conjugated estrogens or Premarin®; 0.25-0.5 mg estradiol), progesterone or a progestin may not be necessary, or might be given in short stretches 3-4 times a year to "bleed off" any tissue that may have accumulated.

Which is better: natural progesterone (oral micronized progesterone or Prometrium) or synthetic progestin (medroxyprogesterone acetate or Provera®); norethindrone (Aygestin®, "NET"), norgestimate, levonogestrel, etc.).

Progesterone, in a usual dose of 200 mg/day (or 100 mg/day, if the estrogen dose is super-low) is "gentler" on the system and causes less adverse effect on lipids, but can cause sleepiness in some and costs a lot more. "Provera®" is the most tested and cheapest, but has a more negative effect on lipids and causes adverse mood symptoms in 5-10% of women. Norgestimate and levonorgestrel are stronger progestins, found in some birth control pills. Norethindrone is somewhere in between. Personal preference. They all work. If you will be taking a progestogen ("natural" progesterone or a progestin) continuously, progesterone or norethindrone are probably preferable over Provera®, although periodic <u>cyclic</u> withdrawal every 3-4 months (if on very low dose estrogen) may be the safest.

## SERMs (SELECTIVE ESTROGEN RECEPTOR MODULATORS)

What can these do? Who should take them?

SERMs are a class of compounds that are not estrogens but are synthesized to "look like estrogen" to the receptors in tissues in different parts of the body, especially bones and, to a lesser extent, the cardiovascular system and lipids.

They can be used <u>in place of</u> (not along with) estrogens and have distinct advantages and disadvantages when compared with estrogens.

Sometimes erroneously referred to as "designer estrogens," SERMs are a class, or type, of medication. The only presently available SERM is raloxifene (or Evista®) but, trust me, many more are in the pipeline.

Raloxifene (and other SERMs) are just as good as estrogens in preventing bone loss. (Some SERMs, like high dose estrogens, actually help build bone at a rate of 2-3% a year without the risk inherent in long term, high dose estrogens).

Raloxifene is as good as estrogen in helping with lipids and protecting the heart. And, as a distinct added bonus, raloxifene has a <u>protective</u> effect on the breasts. It lowers the risk of development of breast cancer. Also, SERMs do not stimulate the endometrium to grow, decreasing the risk of uterine cancer. (As SERMs have no effect on the uterine lining, there's no need to take progesterone or a progestin as a co-therapy).

Additionally, SERMs do not have any of the potential estrogen-related side effects listed earlier in this chapter.

Sounds good, eh? So, what are the downsides? (Nothing in medicine is free!)

Raloxifene in no way helps with the disturbing symptoms of peri-menopause (which is the reason, really, most women elect to take hormones in the first place). There is no evidence either that it aids in vaginal moisture/lubrication or "feelings of well being," skin tone, hair texture, etc.

Presently, SERMs have a definite place in the menopausal replacement/supplementation armamentarium, as we shall see a bit later in this chapter as we unravel the mysteries of hormonal replacement.

<u>However</u>, the world of hormonal supplementation is about to be turned upside down in the next several years with the development and introduction of <u>new SERMs</u> which will not only be bone and breast and uterine protective, but will go a long way toward mitigating disturbing peri-

menopausal symptoms and may have positive effects on libido as well. (see Chapter 18.)

A step closer to the holy grail..

## ALL THE PRESENTLY AVAILABLE TYPES OF ERT/HRT

I.  Oral Estrogens
    1.  Conjugated equine estrogens (Premarin®). The longest used and most researched estrogen. (In fact, virtually all of the long-running studies of hormone replacement have been done utilizing Premarin®, usually at a dose of 0.625 mg (the most common long-term dosage, but not the lowest available).

        Premarin® is truly a "natural product," but not from human sources. It is extracted from the urine of mares who are continually kept in a state of "artificial pregnancy..."
    2.  Esterified conjugated estrogens. This is a synthetic; the same dosages as Premarin®. One of the well studied estrogens.
    3.  Estradiol (Estrace®, Activella®, or Prefest®). A "bioidentical," synthesized from soybeans to mimic estradiol 17-beta, the most common, naturally-occurring estrogen secreted from the ovary. Doses are 0.5 mg, 1 mg and 2 mg.
    4.  Ethinyl estradiol (Estinyl®, FemHRT®). Synthesized. The exact same estrogen that is in all the birth control pills. Long track record. Somewhat "stronger" than the other oral estrogens (so doses are lower).

        These estrogens may be given alone or in combination with progesterone or a progestin.

II. Combined Oral Estrogen/Progestin Products
    1.  PremPro/PremPhase®. Combinations of Premarin® and Provera®, given either continually or cyclicly.
    2.  Activella®; FemHRT®. Combinations of either estradiol or ethinyl estradiol plus norethindrone in low dosages.
    3.  Ortho Prefest. Combination of estradiol and norgestimate, with the progestin given in repeating patterns of 3 days estrogen only, followed by 3 days of estrogen plus progestin, thus minimizing the total amount of progestin while still preventing endometrial buildup within the uterus.

III. Estradiol Transdermal Patches
    The "patch" is worn on the trunk, front or sides, below the breasts, on the abdomen, or hips, and is changed once or twice a week.

There are two types of patches, the "reservoir patch" (Estraderm®), where the estrogen is in a "reservoir," slowly released into the skin, and "matrix patches," where the hormone is uniformly distributed within the plastic polymer adhesive and released into the skin. The same estrogen, estradiol, is utilized within all the patches. The only difference is size, shape, dosage and longevity of the patch. The reservoir patch (Estraderm®) is being phased out.

Brands include:

1. Climera®. The only presently available patch to last one week (the others last 3-4 days). This is an advantage and a disadvantage. The advantage is that you have to change it less often. The disadvantage is that it's bigger and if you have sensitive skin, you are more likely to get a skin reaction when the patch is left in place for 7 days as opposed to 3-4 days. Generics are available (also quite large in size).

2. Alora®, Esclim®, Vivelle®, Vivelle-Dot®, etc. All contain estradiol. Some come in generics. My preference is the Vivelle-Dot® which, dosage for dosage is much smaller: one third the size of all the other patches (the lowest dose Vivelle-Dot® is the size of a "Chicklet®").

IV. Combined Transdermal Patches

One is presently available, the "Combipatch" (containing estradiol and norethindrone). Nice concept and combination but presently available only in a midrange (0.05 mg) estrogen dose (although 2 progestin doses are available). Usually the lower is used, but the higher can be used if there is breakthrough bleeding).

Expect a larger dosage range and more combination patches in the near future.

V. Creams, Gels, Lotions

Individualized hormonal combinations can be made (compounded) by special "compounding" pharmacies. Most mid-sized and large cities have such a pharmacy (none of the larger "chains" compound) and several reputable mail order compounding pharmacies exist nationwide (see Chapters 7 and 20).

A compounding pharmacy can mix the exact desired dose in combination of estriol, estradiol, estrone and progesterone as well as testosterone, DHEA and pregnenolone (the latter two may affect energy levels and may be helpful in the treatment of chronic fatigue—see Chapters 7 and 16).

Since combinations of the estrogens produced by woman's own ovaries (estriol, estrone and estradiol) are the most "physiologic," it may be true that compounded combinations of these estrogens in dosages regulated by your hopefully knowledgeable practitioner, may be better tolerated by sensitive individuals or women who have difficulty with other commercially available hormonal products. Usually a physician or nurse practitioner or naturopath knowledgeable in "complementary and alternative medicine" can help with compounded combinations.

## VI. Injectable Hormones

Sometimes, if all else fails and estrogen therapy is indicated, relief can be obtained by means of a long-acting estrogen injection, every 3-4 weeks.

## VII. Vaginally Absorbed Hormones (low dose)

Estrogen, in the form of low-dose estradiol cream (Estrace®), tablet (Vagifem®) or ring (Estring®), or conjugated estrogen cream (Premarin®), may be applied locally into the vagina and has good effect, after a short while of usage, on increasing vaginal lubrication/moisture, vaginal pliability, and frequently diminishing bladder irritability by estrogenizing the base of the bladder.

The advantage of this method of delivery is that there is extremely little systemic absorption and minimal effect on the uterine lining as well.

The disadvantage is that there is little systemic absorption, so vaginal estrogen administration does not improve other peri-menopausal symptoms, nor does it (for better or for worse) help with cardiac and bone density issues.

It has little effect on breast physiology. A small amount of estrogen (these creams and rings release 0.007-0.15 mg/day) is absorbed, and sensitive women occasionally do have initial breast tenderness.

Cream is the cheapest, and after a short time of usage (1-2 months) is usually effective. The vaginal tablets (Vagifem®) which come with an individual thin plastic applicator are easy to use. The ring (a bit over 2" in diameter; the size of a small diaphragm) is placed in the vagina and contains estradiol in a reservoir in the center of the ring, releasing ±7.5 mcg per day (a microgram is 1/1000th of a mg). It lasts ±3 months and can, if desired, be removed (or not) during lovemaking.

## BRAND NEW:

The first intravaginal estrogen product approved to treat hot flashes as well as the vaginal symptoms of menopause was just released, hitting the market in June/July 2003. It releases therapeutic levels of estrogens.

Called "Femring®," the device is a flexible, self-inserted ring that releases a controlled dose of estradiol acetate over a 3-month period and is available in two dosage strengths: 0.05 mg/day and 0.1 mg/day.

It may be inserted and removed at will, offering potential benefits over daily, twice daily or weekly products for the therapy of moderate to severe hot flashes and symptoms of vulvar atrophy associated with menopause.

## WHICH IS BEST AND WHY:

You know, it's whatever works at the lowest successful dose and only for as long as needed. That said, my bias is definitely for the transdermals (patches or compounded preparations), but let's cover all.

Of the orals, I would tend to go with estradiol over Premarin®. It more closely mimics the body's naturally-occurring estrogen, and seems to have a bit longer half life (lasts longer) than Premarin®, with less nighttime hot flashes. I'd tend to go with the 0.5 mg dose, but 1 mg is OK, although I'd work down to 0.5 mg or lower once symptoms were controlled.

Progesterone? I'd go with norethindrone or micronized progesterone as first choice, but so long as lipids are fine and there are no adverse psychological symptoms, medroxyprogesterone (Provera®) is perfectly satisfactory (at lowest dose).

For long-term use, I'd certainly go with the lowest available dose, preferably a transdermal, either unopposed with regular ultrasound surveillance of the uterine lining, or periodic progesterone withdrawal. A very equally acceptable alternative would be low dose transdermal with daily low dose oral norethindrone or micronized progesterone.

Transdermals are continually released through the skin, leading to less "gaps in coverage" (e.g., breakthrough nighttime hot flashes). There are more dosages of transdermals available. They are easy to use. They bypass the liver and digestive system, leading to less GI symptoms. Unlike oral estrogens, which increase sex hormone binding globulin (SHBG), a blood protein which can diminish free circulating testosterone (and have an adverse effect on libido), transdermal estrogen has no adverse effect on sexual desire. It's also easier to "down-regulate," as discussed below.

How do you down-regulate on the patch? Simple. Once you've "acclimatized" to your patch, slowly (month by month) trim off 10%, then 20%, then 30% of the patch. (You can even self-regulate, cutting off more or less, depending on how you're feeling.) Generally, each lower dose patch is 33⅓ lower than the preceding dose, so when you've "trimmed off" approximately ⅓ of your patch, you are at the next lower commercially available dose!

Downside of patches? Some persons are quite sensitive to the adhesive and get rashes where patches are applied. This sometimes can be mitigated by spraying a macromolecular steroid spray to the skin area just before applying the patch. Also, although patches usually stay on quite well, in some people excessive perspiration, bathing, etc., may loosen the patch.

THE "IDEAL" HORMONE REGIMEN? (Again, remember: you are an individual. What works for your neighbor may not be ideal for you!)

Start high enough to rapidly control symptoms (e.g., 1 mg oral estradiol, 0.625 mg Premarin®, 0.05 mg or more transdermal estradiol patch; BiEst crème 2.5-3.25 mg), working down after 6-12 months of therapy.

For oral estrogens, mix your pill with the next lowest dose and alternate dosages, slowly working down to the next lower dose.

It's easier with the patch. Just trim off a bit. Start with ±10%, going to ±30-35% over a 6-month period of time. As these patches are a matrix of hormones embedded in a plastic polymer (except for Estraderm), nothing is going to "spill out."

Cremes can be compounded to your exact specifications.

Therefore, if you are going to remain on estrogen more than 2 years, by that time you will be on the lowest and safest available dosage regimen.

If you still have your uterus, you will need to take some sort of progesterone or progestin at mid-doses. However, once you are on the lowest estrogen dose, you certainly can get away with a much lower dose of progesterone or progestin and possibly none at all, other than two weeks of progesterone, medroxyprogesterone acetate or norethindrone every 4 months (an ultrasound to rule out any tissue buildup is equally satisfactory, although less cost-effective).

Is all you need increased vaginal lubrication, more support/pliability of the vaginal tissues? In that case, all you may need is low-dose vaginally applied estrogen (see availability above) alone, or in combination with another regimen.

How long should you stay on HRT? Don't necessarily look on HRT as a long-term proposition (although for some individuals it may be). Review your situation and what is new yearly with your (hopefully up-to-date) physician and make an annual decision. This is not something you need to plan long-term when you initiate hormonal supplementation. You are definitely safe with short-term use. So much is changing and new and safer compounds are becoming available, so yearly decisions are the best regarding ongoing usage.

## WEIGHING THE BENEFITS AND RISKS OF HRT: "THE BOTTOM LINE"

There are so many different ways of doing this. Which one works better FOR YOU relating to your symptoms, your family history and personal history, your fears, desires, successes and failures?

Understand, please, that you can traverse peri-menopause and menopause without hormones (and with or without non-hormonal alternatives) and that there is no real need to be on HRT... "forever."

The idea of giving a woman a choice of therapeutic approaches is threatening to those who believe they know what is best for women. The thought that a woman might look at the admittedly inconclusive evidence that we have and come to a conclusion different from the self-proclaimed experts' deeply held belief is anathema.

But that is your goal: Self-determination and the development of the individualized regimen (both short and long term) that WORKS FOR YOU.

I.  SHORT TERM (defined as 2, but probably up to 5 years).

Unless you are one who enjoys a hair coat, there is no need to suffer. Do what is necessary and feels best psychologically to be comfortable. EXERCISE AND A GOOD DIET ARE A MUST IN EVERY REGIMEN.

What are the alternatives?

1.  Soy, herbals, and botanicals only (see next chapter for details).
2.  Hormonal supplementation ("ERT" or "HRT"), via either transdermal or oral administration at the lowest dose that provides symptomatic relief. This may be oral contraceptive pills, if there are no contraindications, and cycle regulation is part of the equation. It may be low dose estrogen only (transdermal or oral) if you are still ovulating and need only something to smooth out the "peaks and valleys." It may be estrogen only if you have no uterus or low dose estrogen only with occasional 10-14 day additions of progesterone or progestin to "bleed off" any tissue that may have formed, or it may be cyclic or continuous estrogen and progesterone/progestin.

    Once symptomatic relief has been obtained, slowly wean down over 6-12 months (it may take longer) to the lowest possible dose (e.g., 0.025 or 0.0375 mg transdermal estradiol patch; 0.25 or 0.5 mg oral estradiol; 0.3-0.45 mg of conjugated estrogens or Premarin® 1.25 mg BiEst creme). At the same time, wean your progesterone/progestin dose down (from 200 mg progesterone down to 100 mg; from 1 mg norethindrone down to 0.5 mg; or from 2.5

Provera® down to 1.25 or 1.5 mg). In fact, the safest (cardiac and breast-wise) may be, when you are down to a low (e.g., 0.0375 or lower patch; 0.5 mg pill) estrogen dose, stop your daily progesterone and go to a 10-14 day 3-6 month "withdrawal" dosing.

3.  If your need is for bone protection only, use alendronate (Fosamax®) or resedronate (Actonel®). (See Chapter 10.)

    If your need is for lipid protection only, use one of the statins (Lipitor®, Mevacor®, etc.). (See Chapter 11)

    If you need bone protection and are high risk for breast cancer, use a SERM (e.g. raloxifene or tamoxifen).

    If you have these needs and have hot flashes and many other symptoms too, add-in non-hormonal substances and maybe herbs and botanicals (see next chapter).

II. LONG TERM (greater than 5 years)

Are there any reasons to be on estrogen supplementation long term? Yes, of course, if your bone density is low. If your "bad" cholesterol is high and there is a family history of heart disease. If vaginal dryness, urinary urgency, dry skin, etc. have been issues.

But is it estrogen that is best in the long term??

There is no evidence that short term estrogen supplementation (defined as up to 2-3 and most likely 5 years) increases cancer risk, and this research is with doses in excess of the present available low dose preparations. Of course, two years would, one suspects, be safer than five. But that short of a time may be impractical in many women.

Now I'm talking of post-menopausal replacement, not peri-menopausal supplementation. Adding a very low dose estrogen while a woman is still cycling just "adds to the pot"; her own endogenous hormones are much stronger than the small amount of estrogen supplementation she is taking to "smooth out the peaks and valleys."

Extrapolating from presently-available data, the increased risk of developing breast cancer by taking post-menopausal estrogen therapy is both dose and time dependent. There appears to be absolutely no increased risk at practically any dosage for two years and no increased risk for up to 4/5 years if on low-dose estrogens. The increased risk of breast cancer, blood clots, and gallbladder disease while taking ultra-low dose estrogens after 5 years is probably no greater than 3-8 additional instances per 10,000 women for breast cancer, "blood clots," and gallbladder disease (coupled with a somewhat diminished risk of colon cancer), in addition to the other effects, beneficial or otherwise, discussed above. This may be a risk some women are willing to take for the aggregate benefits to them of estrogen supplementation.

For more specific information on the relationship of estrogen and breast cancer, see Chapter 9.

## COMPARING APPLES WITH ORANGES: A WORD ABOUT THE "WHI"

The WHI (Women's Health Initiative) study is a large scientific study of many thousands of women. The results from this study, dribbling in over the past year, have served as continual fodder for front-page stories in the print media, and radically changed the thinking of tens of thousands of physicians and millions of patients regarding hormone replacement therapy. What was "hormones forever" is now "hormones never."

The truth, as is so often the case, lies well within these extremes.

We've heard from WHI that, in the study group, hormones not only "cause breast cancer," but "don't protect against heart disease" (and may actually accelerate it). That, in fact, cognition in women taking hormones is worse (more Alzheimer's) and, to add insult to injury, that hormones do not improve peri-menopausal symptoms (hot flashes, mood disturbances, etc.), which is the major reason women start them in the first place.

READ ON!... Let's look at the "fine print."

"In the study group..." Who did the WHI study? Is this group applicable to you (who are now sitting here reading this book).

The average age of women in the WHI is 67 years! This is/was not a study of peri-menopausal women. It is a study of post-menopausal women (most were over 60 when they enrolled). It was a study to determine the long-term cardiovascular effects of estrogens in post-menopausal women. In fact, all women who were peri-menopausal, or newly post-menopausal with symptoms (e.g., hot flashes, insomnia, mood disturbances, etc.) were not accepted in the study. (Since this was a "double blind" study, with some participants receiving hormones and some placebo, the researchers did not want to disadvantage symptomatic peri-menopausal women by giving them a sugar pill.)

It is well known that, in the short term, estrogens are risky in women with preexisting coronary vascular disease, as the slight hemodynamic ("blood flow") change caused by estrogens can increase risks of an adverse event in women with already narrowed blood vessels. Estrogens are known to exert their protective effect long-term (after 10 or more years) by decreasing plaque formation secondary to estrogen's favorable effect on lipids (an effect partially mitigated by the administration of a progestin—especially "Provera®"—but not necessarily bioidentical progesterone or norethindrone.).

So, what did the researchers expect to find in this group of older women in which one would suspect not a small number would have preexisting coronary vascular disease? Of course there was an increase in adverse events in this group, since the study of the combined estrogen and progesterone pills was terminated after only five years, not long enough to begin to see the long-term effects that have been noted in other large, longer-timed studies.

Cognitive effects (read: Alzheimer's)? Again, apples and oranges. Other large studies have shown the protective effect of estrogen on the long-term risk of developing Alzheimer's disease if started at menopause (approximately age 45-55) and continued for 10 years, whereas users who initiated HRT after the age of 60 and continued 5-10 years experienced an increase in their risk of Alzheimer's.

Thus, the study group of WHI would be <u>expected</u> to have these findings since HRT was initiated at an older age and not taken long enough to assess any long-term protective effects.

It is also important to note is that the adverse effects in both the breast (which, by the way, was only slight and not statistically significant) and cardiovascular system were in the study group taking oral estrogen and the relatively potent progestin, Provera®. The group taking <u>estrogen only</u> had no such adverse effects.

As for the finding that "estrogens did not appear to improve symptoms such as hot flashes, mood disturbances, and insomnia," <u>peri-menopausal women with these symptoms were not included</u> in the study (only older and post-menopausal women). One would not <u>expect</u> estrogens to help these symptoms in this group of women who did not have major problems in this area to begin with! Duhhh!

The take-home message? The WHI does not prove short-term estrogen (or estrogen plus bioidentical progesterone or norethindrone) to be unsafe. It does find that giving estrogen (especially estrogen and the progestin medroxyprogesterone, or Provera®) to older women for the purpose of cardio protection or bone loss prevention only is short-sighted.

It also shows that estrogens <u>alone</u> are probably better for breast, cardiovascular system and ??cognition, than estrogen plus continuous progestin.

This makes the case for:

1. Lowest dose estrogen that is effective,
2. Progesterone rather than progestin, if continuous therapy is utilized,
3. Low dose estrogen alone, with periodic (every 3-6 months) progestin or progesterone withdrawal is probably best, and
4. Take estrogen only as long as needed (e.g., 2-3; certainly less than 4-5 years post-menopausally), unless there is a very good reason to continue, and you understand and are willing to accept the small increased risk of a breast malignancy.

## "SUSAN'S STORY"

Susan LaPointe gathered up her reading material, overflowing purse, skirts, and 7-year-old and trotted back to my office. "If my friends knew I was here, I'd be in deep doo-doo. I'm an old hippie," she said, and her lack of makeup, Birkenstocks, and flowing skirts confirmed the fact. "I'm taking dong quai, licorice, wild raspberry, red clover and black cohosh," she exclaimed on her way to the easy chair, "but, really, none of it is working. My teenagers are driving me crazy! My mother-in-law is moving in in 2 weeks and if I don't feel better soon, I may just run away!"

Her 16-year-old son had just gotten his driver's license and her 14-year-old daughter was "high drama" and knew "just where to stick the knife."

"I knew I was going into menopause when my periods started getting irregular when I was maybe 44," she continued. "Last year the hot flashes started getting bad, my memory was in the toilet, and I sure wasn't sleeping good. So I went to 'Nature's Remedies' and Lynn suggested the dong quai and Women's Menopausal Supplement, which has the licorice, wild raspberry, black cohosh and clover extract in it. A couple of my friends take this and say it's all but stopped their flashes 'n stuff. I knew it would take some time, but I've been on this for almost a year and I'm a basket case. I hate to say it, but I think I need <u>something stronger</u>..."

Susan was now 46, right in the middle of the "peri-menopausal curve." She had no particularly increased risk factors for breast cancer or heart disease. Her lipids weren't bad and her blood pressure was normal.

Her last menstrual period was 5 months previously and she had been irregular over the preceding 6-9 months.

We discussed the alternatives. She could continue on her botanicals, perhaps increasing her soy intake, trying to stay away from hot flash "triggers," and working on stress reduction.

After confirming that, in fact, I was <u>not</u> interested in adopting her teens, and not wanting to give up her coffee (which she admitted was a trigger), but which she "couldn't do without," Susan rejected this alternative.

She was, she made clear, "ready for help." Compounding her already stressful family life was the fact that her very high-maintenance mother-in-law was moving in in two weeks. It was this that had prompted her visit. "I need to be mellow by that time or I may kill myself," she said, only half jokingly. "I need hormones."

Additionally, I discovered while completing history taking, her sexual desire had fallen considerably over the preceding year. Although orgasms were still satisfying to her, she could "care less if Paul touched me or not" and this had added an additional dimension of stress.

Since Susan "needed help" relatively quickly and I didn't want to deplete her probably already tenuous level of free testosterone, we decided on a moderate/moderately strong dose of estradiol. We discussed the pros and cons of commercially available estradiol patches vs. compounded estrogen crème combinations. As her insurance did not cover compounded preparations, we decided on a transdermal patch (0.075 mg Vivelle-Dot®). Along with this, I placed Susan on oral micronized progesterone (Prometrium®) 200 mg/day, possibly switching laterally to a compounded preparation if her results were suboptimal, seeing what her menstrual pattern would be over the next few months. I warned her that, with the dose of estradiol and progesterone which would initially lead to some uterine endometrial tissue build-up, and the fact that she might still be occasionally ovulating, she would probably have some irregular bleeding and occasional menses. I gave her a chart to keep track of all bleeding episodes and asked her to return in a month for follow up.

Susan returned 4 weeks later, feeling much better. Her disturbing symptoms "were history" and she'd moved her mother-in-law in "amazingly without incident." She still didn't have much of a sex drive and asked me if she might try testosterone supplementation. We decided on a low dose transdermal lotion (½ cc of micronized testosterone in lotion form, 10 mg per cc strength, starting every night and then falling back to 3-4 times weekly when she was feeling better). I ordered a salivary testosterone level to get a baseline and to help me with follow up, and we discussed a "taper off schedule" to get her down to a more modest 0.05 mg estradiol dose in the next 3-4 months. She would begin by cutting 10% off of the patch, increasing by 5-10% every few weeks until she had cut off a third-this would put her at the next lowest (0.05 mg) dose.

She returned for follow-up 5 months later, in July. She was still on the 0.075 mg patch, she told me, as she experienced a recurrence of symptoms when she tried to taper off. She had had 3 bleeding episodes (2 "like a period"; 1 lighter and shorter) in the preceding 5 months. She had stopped the testosterone as she "didn't need." Her libido had nicely returned as she felt better, less stressed, and was getting more restful sleep.

I told her to try again to begin taper-down (she'd now been on supplementation 6 months) from 0.075 to 0.05, and to keep her progesterone at 200 mg per day to inhibit any possibility of hyperplasia (abnormal tissue buildup) in the uterus.

I plan to see Susan in another 3 months, planning to do a brief ultrasound assessment of the uterine lining at that time to rule out any evidence of excess tissue formation, as well as to see how she's doing on her "taper-down." Hopefully she can maintain on 0.05 within 6 months and then in another 6 months begin to taper-down to 0.0375 (a low but not the lowest dose) at which time I will taper her progesterone to 100 mg/day. If all goes well, she should be down to "super low dose" (0.025 mg) within 2 years.

Susan had a lot of questions regarding how long she would "have to be on this stuff." "One thing at a time," I told her. "There's no hurry. You're not disadvantaging yourself with this short-term estrogen therapy. When you get down to mini doses in a year or three, when you should be fully through menopause, you can decide if you want to stay at that level or taper off altogether. And who knows but that new and better alternatives will probably be available at that time."

*Christian Science is so often therapeutically successful because it lays stress on the patient's believing in his or her own health rather than in Noah's Ark or the Ascension.*
—J.B.S. Haldane, from
"The Duty of Doubt," *Possible Worlds*

# CHAPTER SEVEN

## ALTERNATIVES...ALTERNATIVES... ALTERNATIVES...ALTERNATIVES
### (Herbs, Botanicals, Supplements, Compounded Preparations and other Non-Hormonal Approaches)

Many midlife women seek alternatives to conventional hormone replacement therapy for peri-menopausal symptoms, and are concerned about side effects associated with "conventional" HRT, have fears about breast cancer, concerns over the alleged mistreatment of horses in the production of conjugated estrogens and criticisms about hormones that are not identical to those occurring in nature.

Over $10 billion yearly is spent in purchasing these alternative remedies. What are they? Which work and which do not? How and when to use them and in what dosage? Which combinations work and which may be risky? What "complementary" non-hormonal regimens and lifestyle adaptations enhance quality of life for women as they age?

Physicians' and other health practitioners' information about alternative therapies will increase in coming years, and the growing number of available choices will allow more individualization of treatment.

What is "Natural"?

If you answer "all products that are made in plants," or "native to a living organism (plant and animal)" that is correct. By definition, then, Premarin® (made from pregnant mare's urine) is "...natural."

But where it is natural for the plant, is it natural for the human body? What is it metabolized (changed) into and how does that substance affect the body? How do these substances interact with each other and with other medications the individual happens to be taking? Anything that is being used that is not supported by good unbiased clinical data amounts, for better or for worse, to self-experimentation with one's own body. The fact is that "Premarin®," even in doses far higher than presently used, was previously thought to be "perfectly safe." (It has recently been found to increase the risk of stroke, heart attack, blood clot and breast cancer in older women.)

The term "natural" is little more than an advertising gimmick used to sell everything from hormones to hair care products, from vitamins to vitality enhancers, from garden aids to groceries.

What is "natural"? Is Premarin® natural? What about compounded estriol/estradiol/estrone ("Tri-Est") hormonal cream, or oral or transdermal estradiol patches? Are they natural? The latter, more correctly, are "bioidentical," synthesized in the lab from a plant source (in this case, soybeans), to mimic the molecule found "...in nature."

Are soy or red clover-derived isoflavones—"natural"? More correctly, these are phytoestrogens, plant-sourced material that, although not an estrogen, has estrogen-like activities.

Are black cohosh, evening primrose oil or chasteberry "natural"? More correctly, they are botanicals, derived from plant sources.

Let's call a spade a spade! "Natural" is a confusing term meant to soothe the public into buying a particular product (or going to a particular practitioner). Better to use the terms "bioidentical," "phytoestrogen," and "herb" or "botanical."

There is, as yet, very little research comparing the relative safety and efficacy of many of these supplements to the conventional regimens of, say, conjugated equine estrogens and medroxyprogesterone (PremPro®). There is nothing that I can see to suggest they are unsafe—it is simply that their safety is unknown. *Caveat emptor*—let the buyer beware.

## EXERCISE, DIETARY AND LIFESTYLE MODIFICATIONS

There is no free lunch. WHATEVER you decide, whichever choice you make regarding hormones, no hormones, herbs, botanicals or other alternatives, you can't sit on the couch watching TV, sipping beer and eating bonbons and expect to feel good and be healthy.

The different experiences of menopause in different cultures may, in part, be due to diet and lifestyle. A high-fiber diet decreases the risk of cardiovascular diseases, a low-fat diet improves the cholesterol profile, and an anti-oxidant-rich diet and increased intake of soy products may diminish hot flashes and other menopausal symptoms.

Several lifestyle approaches may help in the management of menopausal symptoms. Smoking cessation diminishes the risk of cardiovascular disease and osteoporosis, and may cut down on hot flashes. Low alcohol intake also diminishes hot flashes and osteoporosis risk. Maintaining regular sexual activity may help with vaginal dryness and improve depressive symptoms ("use it or lose it"). Regular exposure to sunlight may help depressive symptoms and decrease risk of osteoporosis. Relaxation and stress reduction also diminish the risk of cardiovascular disease and may improve depressive symptoms. Hot flashes may be improved by avoiding getting too hot and paying attention to "triggers" (the things you have found that initiate your symptoms).

Exercise is of paramount importance. Don't exercise to lose weight. Exercise to be healthy, sleep and feel better, and generally be happier.

Exercise is not something you have to like. It's like a job you "have to do" to put food on the table. You HAVE to exercise to feel and be healthy!

I'm talking of 30-45 minutes (or more) of "out of breath, sweaty" and occasional weight-bearing exercise at least 4-5 times per week.

Aerobics, power walking, cycling, running/jogging, swimming, at-home or health club machines, active sports such as singles tennis, basketball, volleyball, etc. are all good. Out-of-breath sweaty exercise. Plan on setting aside 45-60 minutes every day, so if you miss here and there you won't feel bad. (If you end up only having 15-20 minutes, this is still better than nothing!)

## VITAMINS AND MINERALS

1.  Calcium, magnesium, and vitamin D

Whatever treatment is used to prevent and treat osteopenia / osteoporosis (osteopenia is a milder, precursor of osteoporosis), it is essential to provide adequate dietary supplemental calcium and vitamin D.

Approximately 30 minutes in full sunlight per day supplies adequate vitamin D. Supplementing 400-800 I.U. per day is recommended for women who do not receive sun exposure. In the United States, ±400 I.U. of vitamin D is added to each cup of milk, yogurt, etc. It is included also in most vitamin and mineral supplements.

Calcium requirements are approximately 1000-1500 mg per day. Dietary sources are important (see Chapter 10). Or, you can get it in pill form.

Adequate magnesium in the ratio of approximately 1:2 with calcium may also be helpful for bone health. An intake of approximately 600 mg per day should be sufficient.

2.  Vitamin E

Vitamin E at a dose of 400-800 I.U. per day may play a role in prevention of atherosclerosis (hardening of the arteries) by lowering blood lipids. At this or higher doses (800-1200 mg per day) vitamin E can help decrease hot flashes in many peri-menopausal women.

3. <u>Vitamins B6, B12 and Folic Acid</u>

Supplementing with various B vitamins may be a helpful addition for reduction of osteopenia and cardiovascular disease.

Milk, milk products and red meat are converted into homocysteine (a blood protein which has adverse effects on blood vessels and the heart), which requires adequate levels of B6, B12 and Folic acid to metabolize into harmless amino acids. If this doesn't occur, homocysteine levels rise. Elevated homocysteine is as dangerous as smoking as a risk factor for cardiovascular disease. (Estrogen, by the way, also helps control homocysteine levels.)

## DIETARY SUPPLEMENTS: HERBS, BOTANICALS, PHYTOESTROGENS

So-called alternative approaches to menopause are used so widely that it might be more accurate to consider HRT as the true alternative medicine! Nearly half of all menopausal women use complementary therapies including vitamins, herbs, and soy products to help treat their symptoms. Around 20% of these use complementary or alternative therapies alone and approximately 25% use "conventional" and "alternative" methods (compared with 20% who use HRT only).

The decision to use an alternative is not so much dissatisfaction with conventional treatment, but that many women regard the complementary agents as more in keeping with their own philosophy of health and life.

1. <u>Herbs and Botanicals</u>

Almost half of the drugs commonly used today are either plant products or phytochemicals (plant chemicals that are helpful to human health) that were initially isolated from plants but are now synthesized by chemical processing techniques and are called "bioidenticals."

Plants are used therapeutically in the form of herbs, oils, pills, teas or tinctures.

§ <u>Bulk Herbs</u> are raw or dried plants used as powders or pulvers (ultra-fine powders) to make teas or tinctures. The powder can also be put into a capsule or compounded into tablet form.

§ <u>Oils</u> are concentrates of fat-soluble chemicals from herbs, concentrated and used externally.

§ <u>Tablets or capsules</u> may be compounded for exact dosage and ease of use.

§ <u>Tinctures</u> are alcohol-extracted concentrates usually added to water or placed directly into the mouth or under the tongue.

§ <u>Teas</u> are used to extract solubles from the herb by adding hot water. The potency is determined by steeping time.

While the word "herbal" refers to only leaves and stems of plants, the term "botanical" also denotes foods and supplements derived from any part of the plant, including seeds, flowers, fruits and roots.

## BLACK COHOSH

A member of the buttercup family, black cohosh (folk names include *black snake root* and *bug bane*) has a long history in folk medicine, especially among Native Americans, who boiled the root in water and drank the tea to treat painful menses, labor pains, upset stomach and arthritis. Extracts of black cohosh have been used in Germany for over 60 years and are well studied in the German literature, which seems to show that black cohosh binds to estrogen receptors. There appears to be no contraindications to the use of black cohosh.

Black cohosh is the main ingredient in Lydia Pinkham's Vegetable Compound and in extracts sold over the counter as *Remifemin®* here and in Europe.

Several studies have shown a significant improvement in hot flashes, with reductions of 50-75%, while others have shown black cohosh to be no more effective than placebo.

The dosage is 40 drops of the extract (or two 20 mg tablets) twice daily. Side effects aren't common, but occasionally include gastric discomfort. Dizziness, headaches, and tremors have been noted.

## RED CLOVER

Red clover, a plant that contains the phytoestrogens formonentin, biochainin, diadzein and genistein, was originally used by Native Americans to treat whooping cough, gout, and cancer.

Scientific studies have yielded mixed results. While some studies have failed to demonstrate that red clover extract was more effective than placebo in decreasing hot flashes, others found that women who took 40 mg per day (the recommended dose), experienced a significant reduction in their hot flashes.

Red clover was removed from the USP formulary in 1946 because of supposed ineffectiveness. However, Promensil®, a red clover derivative, exerts its effects through concentrated levels of isoflavones synthesized from the plant, and seems to have a generally positive, if irregular, effect on hot flash symptoms.

It is possible that the 40 mg dose (used in most studies) is ineffective for many women who require a higher dosage (up to 80 mg per day). This may be the reason for poor results in some studies.

Like many other herbal and botanical products, red clover takes 2-3 months to be effective. Its possible estrogenic effects have not been studied.

## EVENING PRIMROSE

Native Americans ate the leaves, roots, and seed pods for food and made extracts to treat a variety of conditions. Today, the flowers and seeds are pressed to make oil that is high in gammalinoleinic acid and omega-6 fatty acids.

Although there are a number of studies in which evening primrose oil has been used successfully to treat eczema and other conditions, it appears to have no benefit over placebo for hot flashes. Studies using evening primrose oil for cyclic breast tenderness have shown inconsistent results.

Evening primrose oil contains several anticoagulant substances and should be used with care by persons at risk for bleeding or those already on anticoagulants.

## ST. JOHN'S WORT

Extracts from this flower have been used for centuries to treat mild depression. The constituents include hypericin, pseudo-hypericin and flavinoids.

Commercial preparations should be standardized to 0.3% hypericin or 0.5% hyperfiren. The recommended dosage is 300 mg of the plant extract as a tablet 3 times a day.

Side effects are similar to (but far less than) those of standard antidepressant medications, including dry mouth, dizziness, and constipation.

## GINKGO BILOBA

This herb is reported to have a wide range of effects, including improvement of memory and slowing of age-associated cognitive decline by enhancing blood flow and oxygen delivery to the brain.

While there are no clear data that ginkgo affects mood, it may be helpful in treating sexual dysfunction associated with prescription antidepressants.

Ginkgo products are standardized for flavone glycoside content at 24% and terpene lactone content at 6%. The usual dose is 60 mg twice daily, although this dose can be doubled in 6-8 weeks if the lower dose is ineffective.

Because it has anticoagulant effects, it should not be used in conjunction with aspirin or prescription anticoagulants. Also, since ginkgo biloba has synergistic effects with vitamin E, caution should be used before taking it with high doses of vitamin E.

## DONG QUAI

Dong Quai, a type of angelica, is the most commonly prescribed Chinese herbal medication for "female problems" and supposedly regulates and balances menstrual cycle and is said to "strengthen the uterus." It is said to exert estrogenic activities.

Although some women report improvement in their hot flashes, scientific studies have not verified that effect. In China it is sold as part of a mixture that includes several other herbs, compared to America where it is sold as a single herb. This may explain its diminished effect in U.S. studies.

Since Dong Quai contains substances which can interfere with blood clotting it should not be used with other anticoagulants. As it is potentially photosensitizing, there is concern that Dong Quai may increase the risk of sun-exposure-related skin cancers.

## VALERIAN ROOT

The common valerian or garden heliotrope has been used traditionally as a tranquilizer or sleep aid. Its effective constituent is thought to be a gamma aminobutyric acid (GABA) derivative. A similar compound has been found in chamomile (also used as a sleep aid).

When taken as an extract, tea or tincture, it seems to provide some mild sedating and calming effects and is frequently used as a natural sleep aid.

Patients should seek products that document valerianic acid content per dosage unit and aim for between 300-600 mg of standardized extracts. It is best taken one hour before going to bed.

It has no known contraindications, but elderly patients (over 70/75) should begin with lower doses.

## LICORICE

Licorice is one of a number of botanicals including ginseng, fenugreek, sarsaparilla, gotu kola, wild yam, and dong quai, which claim (but have not been proven) to have estrogen-like activities.

## SAW PALMETTO

This plant has minor estrogen-like activity (1/10,000th that of estrogen), although a purified extract may have much higher activity. Its use in menopause to stimulate libido is unproven.

## CHASTEBERRY

Chasteberry (or vitex) has been recommended by some for vaginal dryness, menopause and also for depression. It contains some progesterone hormone-like substances (flavenoids and glycosides) and as such may help with the symptoms of depression and breast tenderness with PMS when taken in the second half of the cycle.

The usual dosage for control of PMS is 20 mg of extract daily; symptomatic improvement should be achieved within 3 months.

## GINSENG

There are many types of ginseng—Siberian, Korean, American, white and red. All are called "adaptogens," which help one cope with stress and supposedly boost immunity. Unfortunately, little objective evidence exists that supports claims for its antioxidant and aphrodisiac effects or its ability to improve athletic performance.

Ginseng root, because of its estrogenic properties, can cause vaginal bleeding and breast discomfort. CAUTION: Because ginseng, as sold, is often combined with bee products, susceptible individuals may have allergic reactions.

## WILD YAM

Yam extracts, tablets and cream claim to be progesterone substitutes and are touted as a natural source of DHEA. Sterol extracts from the plant are used by compounding pharmacists as precursors in the biosynthesis of progesterone, DHEA and some other steroids. Mexican yam extract itself is estrogenic, containing the plant sterol diosgenin, an estrogen-like substance.

Natural progesterone is touted as a remedy for peri-menopausal and menopausal symptoms. Recently progesterone cream has been examined in scientific trials. Although no protective effect on bone density has been noted at the dosages tested, significant improvements in hot flashes were. In proper doses, it can be used as a substitute for orally administered progestins or progesterone in the prevention of uterine cancer in women taking hormone replacement therapy.

## KAVA KAVA

This herb has been used for centuries in the South Pacific as an anxiety-reliever, relaxant and sedative. Menopausal patients may take it to aid sleep and reduce anxiety. There are no specific contraindications but caution should be used if you are taking Valium®, Xanax®, etc., or with use along with alcohol.

The Kava product should be standardized to 70 mg of kava lactones per capsule and the daily dose should be in the range of 140-220 mg of kava lactones. Most patients find 1-2 capsules at night before bed is effective.

## PHYTOESTROGENS

Phytoestrogens are naturally occurring compounds found in plants which can exert effects similar to estrogen. They are classified into three groups:

§ Isoflavones (especially genistein and daidzein) are plant sterols found in soy, garbanzo beans and other legumes (beans) as well as red clover.

§ Lignans are a component of the cell wall of plants and are bioavailable as the result of the effect of intestinal bacteria on grains. The highest amounts are found in seed oils, especially flax seed.

§ High concentrations of coumestans are found in red clover, sunflower seeds and bean sprouts.

Phytoestrogens have a variety of activities: estrogenic, anti-estrogenic, anti-oxidant, anti-mutagenic, anti-hypertensive, anti-inflammatory and anti-proliferative (anti-cancer), at least in experimental animals.

The role of phytoestrogens has stimulated interest because those cultures consuming diets high in isoflavones, such as Japanese and Chinese, have a lower incidence of hot flashes, cardiovascular diseases and breast, colon, uterine and prostate cancers when compared to that in westernized countries.

Asian diets typically contain 40-60 mg of isoflavones per day, where American diets are less than 3 mg per day. Westernized diets tend to increase the exposure of tissues to circulating estrogens, thus increasing rates of breast, colon and uterine cancers and maximizing adverse symptoms when these levels fluctuate and then fall during peri-menopause and then menopause.

High soy and high bean food diets may not only lower cancer risk by modifying hormone metabolism and limiting cancer cell growth, but also provide large amounts of fiber, which modifies the level of sex hormones by increasing gastrointestinal motility.

However you slice them, soy and beans are good stuff! The only down sides are occasional bloating and flatulence.

## DHEA

DHEA (dihydroepiandrosterone), sometimes called "the mother hormone," is a substance made in humans by the adrenal glands (located on top of the kidneys) and is available over-the-counter without prescription. It is purported to have energy-enhancing and both estrogen and androgen (male hormone)-like effects. However, the long term effects and proper doses of DHEA still need to be identified.

Preliminary studies have shown that DHEA increases bone density, improves immune function, decreases total cholesterol (as well as the good HDLs) and increases the ability of the body to process sugar. However, even at a dose of only 25 mg per day (recommended dose is 25 mg once-twice per day, although some women take much higher) significantly increased patient levels of both testosterone and estrogen are noted. These increases may be the reason for DHEA's purported effects on bone density and energy levels.

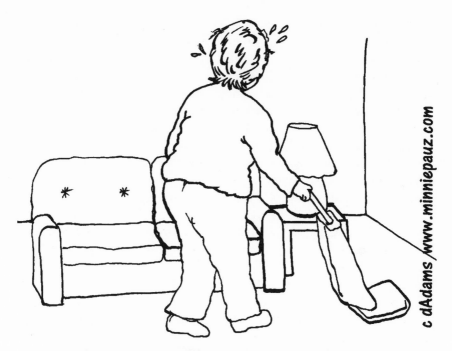

c dAdams /www.minniepauz.com

## There's nothing like soy protein to help power household appliances!

### WHAT'S PROVEN AND WHAT'S NOT?

Limited scientific information about botanicals is available in English, although several new studies are ongoing. Several publications from Europe and Asia give confusing results.

1. Soy/isoflavones. Based on limited studies, the use of soy probably does have benefits in reducing hot flashes.
2. Black cohosh. Also based on limited evidence, black cohosh appears to have a positive effect on sleep disorders, mood disturbance and hot flashes without evidence of toxicity.
3. Evening primrose. Large-scale analyses of the scientific trials of evening primrose oil failed to show improvement in hot flashes beyond those seen with placebo. <u>But</u>, it is not harmful. It works for some people. If it does for you: go for it.
4. Ginseng. Although no differences have been found in improvement of vasomotor symptoms (hot flashes), significant improvements have been noted in "quality of life measures" such as fatigue, depression, general health and well-being. No studies have documented effects on libido in women.

5.  Dong Quai. There's no evidence that dong quai taken alone produces lessening of hot flashes. However, dong quai is never employed in Chinese medicine as an isolated intervention, and herbalists and naturopaths correctly argue that botanicals must be taken together in a "balanced formula" as therapeutic outcome requires the proper joint synergistic action to take place between components.

    A recent study has shown increased growth of MCF-7 (a human breast cancer cell line) in women taking dong quai and ginseng, while black cohosh and licorice root do not have this effect.

6.  St. John's Wort. Many studies have noted that St. John's Wort hypericin produces improvement in mild to moderate depression and possibly seasonal affective disorder ("winter depression").

7.  Valerian Root. Based on existing studies, there is little evidence that valerian improves sleep beyond placebo. But some of my patients say that it works for them.

8.  Chasteberry (or vitex, the chasteberry extract). Although vitex's supposed anti-hormonal activity is the basis for advising its use in treating mastalgia (tender breasts), claims of efficacy are poorly documented. Other trials have shown significant improvements in mood alteration, anger, headache and breast fullness. However, other menstrual symptoms like bloating remain unchanged.

9.  Wild and Mexican Yam. Based on the lack of bioavailability, the hormones in wild and Mexican yam would not be expected to have any efficacy; wild yam extracts are neither estrogenic or progestational.

    Many wild yam extract products contain no yam, but some are laced with progesterone (natural or synthetic) and it is maybe these, rather than the yam itself, which exerts its purported progesterone-like effects in therapy of menopausal and menstrual disorders.

    *This is separate from the <u>bioidentical preparations</u> that are <u>synthesized</u> from yam products by compounding pharmacists.*

Understanding all of this, "natural" is not necessarily an assurance of safety or efficacy, and potentially dangerous drug-herb interactions may occur.

Lack of standardization of botanicals may result in variability of content and efficacy from batch-to-batch and between manufacturers. Lack of quality control and regulation may result in contamination, adulteration or potential misidentification of plant products. Errors in compounding may result in toxic outcome in custom-blended herbal preparations.

Botanicals should not be taken in larger than recommended doses or for longer than recommended duration.

## ALTERNATIVE THERAPIES FOR HOT FLASHES

"Vasomotor instability" (hot flashes) is one of the first and most prominent signs of menopause and can last for several years. "Flashes" are linked to estrogen withdrawal and not just low estrogen levels. The change in the core regulatory temperature control center in the brain sets up the situation where, in susceptible women, even subtle changes in temperature can precipitate a hot flash.

Although the mainstay of menopause-related symptom management has been the use of HRT, there are many women who discontinue hormones due to side effects or who do not want to start in the first place because of fears of cancer and a generalized apprehension of hormones.

It is important to note that in almost all of the placebo-controlled studies (see also Chapter 13) of hot flashes, the placebo groups experienced an approximately 20-30% reduction in hot flashes and this placebo response should be kept in mind by those evaluating the effectiveness of any given intervention.

So: that said—what works??

1.  Vitamins and plant products:

Vitamin E in doses of 800-1200 mg per day reduces hot flashes slightly more than placebo. Vitamin E is inexpensive, nontoxic, and readily available without a prescription. (Women on "blood thinners" should not take high doses of vitamin E.)

The debate over the use of soy for hot flashes continues. Several small studies indicate that 80-120 mg of soy isoflavones per day have a positive effect, while others suggest a lack of beneficial effect.

Soybeans contain 1-2 mg of isoflavones per gram of soy products (28 gms = 1 oz). Not all soy protein products contain isoflavones, however. Some soy powders and capsules are processed with an alcohol extract that removes the isoflavones. In order to ensure that you are receiving the desired dose of isoflavones from a "soy supplement," be certain to ascertain its "isoflavone content."

Outside of Germany, there is a dearth of research on black cohosh for hot flash management. It may be helpful in reducing hot flashes; it probably helps in reducing sweating.

2.  Behavioral Interventions

Sipping cool drinks, avoiding spicy foods and alcohol, having good room air circulation, reducing stress (via paced respiration and relaxation exercises) all help.

3.  Newer antidepressants and other psychoactive medications

The best studied and arguably most effective non-hormonal hot flash intervention in the United States is a newer antidepressant called venlafaxine (Effexor®) in a dose ±37.5 mg once-twice per day.

Other antidepressants such as <u>fluoxetine</u> (Prozac®), <u>citralopram</u> (Celexa®), <u>serataline</u> (Zoloft®) and others in their category may help as well.

<u>Gabepentin</u> (Neurontin®), an anticonvulsant drug frequently used by psychiatrists in the treatment of depression and bipolar disorder, may be a good second-line therapy for women with moderate to severe flashes that don't respond to vitamin E, behavior modifications and other agents.

4. <u>Older Agents</u>

<u>Bellergal-SR®</u> (a combination of belladonna alkaloids and pheno-barbital) has a long history of use for hot flashes, but good clinical data to support its use is limited.

<u>Clonidine®</u> (usually used as a transdermal patch) has been shown to surpass placebo (but not by much) in the reduction of hot flashes, but may have side effects of insomnia, mouth dryness, and constipation.

5. <u>Progesterone and Progestins</u>

Progesterone creme (¼-½ cc of 3-5% creme) or lotion (25-100 mg) massaged into soft skin at bedtime helps with hot flashes in a large percentage of women.

<u>Medroxyprogesterone acetate</u>, usually used in large doses in injectable (or "depo") form, appears to reduce hot flashes to a degree similar to that of estrogen. This is the same medication (DepoProvera®) used as an injectable contraceptive, but in treating hot flashes is given in higher doses (±500 mg) every 2 weeks for 3-4 doses.

A related progestin, megestrol acetate (Megace®), used to treat uterine cancer, is also useful in diminishing flashing, in a dose of 40 mg per day.

## NATUROPATHY, HOMEOPATHY, AND COMPOUNDING; SALIVARY TESTING

This certainly can be a topic for a whole book, and indeed there are several <u>excellent</u> ones already written (see *Discover your Menopause Type* by Joseph Collins, ND).

A thorough treatment of these topics is beyond the scope of this book. Suffice it to say that these modalities are an excellent and generally safe way of treatment.

(As stated elsewhere in this book, THERE ARE MANY SHOES THAT FIT!)

Naturopathy involves treating the <u>whole person</u> (not just "giving a medication" to treat a certain situation). It involves nurturing self-care (via proper nutrition and body awareness), the use of herbal remedies (only a small portion of which are already discussed in this chapter), glandular extracts (preparations of specific tissues or glands from animal sources, used to restore health and function to the tissue or gland targeted) and compounded preparations.

A naturopathic approach to peri-menopausal and menopausal supplementation involves ascertaining each woman's specific "menopause type," if you will, and designing therapy along her individual lines, using the products described above. It in large part involves both the avoidance of substances with anti-estrogenic, anti-progestogenic, and/or anti-androgenic activities and the compounding of specific hormonal creams, lozenges or oral preparations to treat the estrogen loss, progesterone loss, androgen loss, combinations thereof, or hormonal dominance situations that may be present.

A good compounding pharmacist and follow-up, especially with salivary hormone testing, is essential in this mode of therapy.

Compounding and Compounding Pharmacies

Compounding pharmacists are specially-trained pharmacists who prepare customized medications (including bioidenticals) that are designed to the unique needs of each woman.

Upon receiving a prescription or consulting directly with a physician and/or the patient, the pharmacist takes the necessary ingredients (frequently bioidenticals derived from plant sources) and compounds (or blends) them to meet the specific needs of the individual.

There are approximately 2500 compounding pharmacies in the United States (compared to ±40-50,000 "regular" pharmacies). You can locate a compounding pharmacist in your area by contacting the International Academy of Compounding Pharmacists at (800) 927-4227; FAX (281) 495-0602, or www.iacprx.org; or Professional Compounding Centers of America at (800) 331-2498 (www.pccarx.com).

Compounded preparations can include estriol, estradiol, estrone, progesterone, testosterone, DHEA, pregnenolone, and others. Dosage forms can include creams, lotions, special gels to aid in skin penetration, lozenges, pills and capsules.

The down side of compounding is that many times this specific a treatment is not needed, as well as expense (many compounded products are not covered by insurance).

Salivary Testing

The problem with blood testing for hormone levels (other than testing for testosterone and "free testosterone" blood levels, which can be helpful in determining the need for testosterone supplementation) is that hormone levels in the blood change practically "moment to moment" and there is such a broad range of normality (which can differ from individual to individual).

Much of the hormonal and non-hormonal therapeutic approaches in menopause are symptoms-based and empirical. So long as you are doing no harm ("*primum non nocere*") and are using an individualized and common sense approach, relief of symptoms alone can be a good endpoint.

However, if you wish to be a bit more scientific and accurate, salivary tests may be used to measure hormone levels and monitor effects of therapy and, as such, measurements are recommended every 6 months until hormonal levels are stable.

By a relatively new technology, hormone levels can be measured in saliva. These appear to have a consistent relationship to the levels in the blood. Salivary tests are easy to perform, as all you need to do is "spit into a jar" at home, usually 12-24 hours after your last dose of hormones) and mail it into the lab.

There are salivary tests for the different estrogens, progesterone, testosterone, as well as other hormones such as cortisol and DHEA.

Pregnenalone is best measured in the blood, although salivary progesterone levels seem to parallel pregnenalone.

It's probably best for women who take specifically-compounded hormones or hormone precursors such as DHEA, pregnenolone or androstenedione to be evaluated regularly.

Homeopathy

Homeopathy is recognized in 28 different countries all over the world and over 70 different homeopathic remedies (animal, herbal or mineral) have been used with clinical success in women with menopausal discomforts.

Homeopathy involves the use of microdoses of substances, usually in combination, to alleviate symptoms. Some of the basic homeopathics included in multi-homeopathic remedies for menopausal hot flashes symptoms include sepia, carbonate of lime, sachesis (bush master), phosphorus, pulsatilla (wind flower), sanguinaria (blood root), and sulfur.

## The Menopause Symptom Index (MENSI)

Name_____ Date_____

| EXPERIENCE | No | Occasionally | Yes | Is this a problem for you? | |
|---|---|---|---|---|---|
| Hot or warm flushes? | 0 | 1 | 2 | Y | N |
| Palpitations? | 0 | 1 | 2 | Y | N |
| Headaches? | 0 | 1 | 2 | Y | N |
| Sleep disturbances? | 0 | 1 | 2 | Y | N |
| Chest pressure or pain? | 0 | 1 | 2 | Y | N |
| Shortness of breath? | 0 | 1 | 2 | Y | N |
| Numbness? | 0 | 1 | 2 | Y | N |
| Weakness or fatigue? | 0 | 1 | 2 | Y | N |
| Pain in bone joint? | 0 | 1 | 2 | Y | N |
| Memory loss? | 0 | 1 | 2 | Y | N |
| Anxiety? | 0 | 1 | 2 | Y | N |
| Depression? | 0 | 1 | 2 | Y | N |
| Fear of leaving home? | 0 | 1 | 2 | Y | N |
| Loss of urinary control? | 0 | 1 | 2 | Y | N |
| Vaginal dryness? | 0 | 1 | 2 | Y | N |
| Loss of sexual desire? | 0 | 1 | 2 | Y | N |
| Pain with intercourse? | 0 | 1 | 2 | Y | N |
| Disrupted function: Home? | 0 | 1 | 2 | Y | N |
| Disrupted function: Work? | 0 | 1 | 2 | Y | N |

Other symptoms?

MENSI score: (0-38) _____    Number of "Yes" answers: _____

**"CARING FOR WOMEN"  Michael Goodman, MD  (530) 753-2787**
**FAX: (530) 750-0221**

## DIANE'S STORY

As I accompanied Diane back to my office, I discovered that a friend of hers (and patient of mine) had recommended my services. As I usually do, shortly after we'd introduced ourselves and gotten comfortable, I asked Diane what she wished to accomplish by our work together. "To feel a little better," she answered. "Better sleep; a bit more energy."

Although on first appraisal it appeared as if Diane's symptoms were actually quite mild, as we further explored her situation, it became apparent that more was bothering her than she'd first let on.

While her periods were mostly normal, she was increasingly bothered over the preceding six months by both hot flashes and night sweats, and wasn't sleeping well. "I'm waking up tired," she sighed.

We talked about quality REM sleep, and how the temperature regulatory center in her brain was reacting to her ovary's shifts in estrogen production. It was no wonder that the problem that bothered her most was fatigue.

But it was more than that. Although not impacting her professional or home life, she was noting very occasional memory difficulties "...in finding the right word."

"None of these things by themselves are major," she confided. "But when they're all added together, they certainly impact my life."

As we went on in my history taking, I discovered that Diane had just been faced with the heart-wrenching decision to institutionalize her mother who, at age 68, was significantly afflicted with Alzheimer's disease, which had apparently started when she was newly menopausal at age 50. Diane was now 45.

Diane's major issue, it seemed, was worry about "what was to come," uncertainty about how it would effect her, and fear that she'd end up like her mother.

Coupled with this was Diane's stated goal to do as much as possible "...naturally... without medications."

After a brief discussion of ovarian physiology, production of hormones in the ovaries and elsewhere, and what was beginning to normally and naturally happen to her body, we settled down to talk of alternatives. I took note of Diane's stated objective to proceed as "naturally as possible" and asked what that meant to her.

"Well, I don't want to take any hormones," she responded. I explained the difference between botanicals which, although derived from a very natural product (soy beans), was synthesized to exactly mimic the ovary's natural estradiol and therefore function like a hormone, with similar effects.

I compared this with phytoestrogens, directly from plant sources (especially soy and red clover derivatives) and botanicals such as black cohosh, licorice, chasteberry fruit, etc., which were known to have some mediating effects on disturbing mood symptoms, and ginkgo biloba which, because of its mild blood vessel dilating effects, was thought to have some effect on increasing cerebral blood flow and perhaps helping to prevent memory deterioration. We discussed the fact that none of these preparations were known to mediate or prevent the effects of Alzheimer's disease, but that estrogens (especially in individuals with a strong family history) might help in this area.

I noted that, while Diane used to bicycle or walk 4-5 times a week, lately it was down to once or twice. She'd gained 10 lbs. in the past year, a fact that did not set well with her. "I should add weight to my list also," she sighed.

We then settled down to outlining a "first line" regimen.

"First and foremost," I explained, "are some lifestyle changes." We spoke of various hot flash triggers (in Diane's case, alcohol, spicy foods, and hair dryers) and their avoidance. We talked of endorphins and brain serotonin metabolism and outlined an "inviolable" exercise regimen. Diane had a health club membership which she seldom used. Monday, Wednesday and Fridays she would go in before work for 20 minutes of aerobics plus 20 minutes of floor exercises with weights. On Sunday morning she had her regular bike ride with some friends. She assured me she would increase the distance to at least 10 miles, working toward 20. "And one other day as well," I emphasized. "At least 4-5 days per week."

Diane was already pretty savvy about soy. I taught her how to determine isoflavone content of various products, and suggested a supplement of 60-100 mg per day. She would add in ginkgo 60 mg twice daily as well as vitamin E 400 mg in the morning and 800 mg at bedtime. (I warned her not to take aspirin with this combination.)

We both agreed that her energy drain was most likely the result of poor sleep and that a "fatigue workup" wasn't warranted at this time. ("If nothing is helping and your fatigue is worse, we'll revisit this later," I explained.) I gave Diane my little pamphlet on "stress reduction" and a "bedtime ritual" consisting of no alcohol or caffeine within 4 hours of sleep time, 15-30 minutes of meditation and a soothing bath with perhaps a warm beverage just prior to sleep. We talked of Kava Kava and Valerian as additional aid, if needed. Diane chose not to start on any other botanicals at the present time.

"This will take awhile to be effective," I warned, and set up a 6-week appointment to check progress. Before Diane left, she filled out a "MENSI" (Menstrual Symptom Index) so that we could objectively follow her progress (see sample).

At follow-up, Diane was marginally better. Although her occasional memory glitches and daytime hot flashes were still occurring, she was noting better sleep quality and energy. The daytime flashes were the greatest problem.

Additional isoflavones in the form of promensil (a red clover derivative) were added in, and I chided Diane for her lack of establishing an exercise routine. ("You don't have to <u>like</u> it," I reminded her, "you just have to <u>DO IT</u>—if you want to feel better, that is.") I encouraged her in all the areas we were working on and told her to make an appointment in 2 months, or sooner if needed.

She returned in July. Even though the weather had heated up quite a bit, she was happy. "It's not perfect," she said, "but it's very livable."

I had Diane fill out another questionnaire. Where her total score for problem areas had been 16 (with 7 "yes" answers), it was now down to 9 with only 2 yes's.

I spoke briefly of other available options should conditions deteriorate. "There are lots of shoes," I reminded her. "Don't let yourself get crazy if things change. There's always a way to safely work things out."

Diane was happy. "Now," she said, "since I'm doing better, maybe we can work on why I have the sex drive of a banana slug."

And...onward to Chapter 8!!

*Sex is one of the nine reasons for reincarnation...the other eight are unimportant.*

—Henry Miller in *Big Sur and the Oranges of Hieronymus Bosch*

# CHAPTER EIGHT

## SEX!?
## "I Couldn't Care Less...(And I'm Dry to Boot)"

"A woman's sexuality is a journey...always changing, never static. Sexual desires and responses ebb and flow, shifting with adolescence, young adulthood, marriage or life with a partner, pregnancy, child rearing, menopause and aging. Sexuality is always there, in one form or another."

This quote begins a chapter of a wonderful book on women's sexuality[1], a "must read" for women experiencing difficulties not only in the peri-menopause.

There are few things in life that are fun...and free. Sex is one of them. So it makes all the sense in the world for a woman to empower herself to get what she wants, to be where she wants, in comfortable alignment in her sexual universe.

The goal (not too dissimilar from the goal at other times of life) is to be comfortable, unconflicted, pleased, satisfied and, if applicable, in synchrony with your mate.

That is the goal of this chapter: to help you achieve that state.

Since this is a book on midlife, the sexual issues and their solutions discussed herein relate mostly to the peri- and post-menopause.

### MIDLIFE SEXUAL ISSUES AND THEIR RESOLUTION

What are the sexual issues that I see women bring with them into my office? They fall into several categories:

1. DESIRE ISSUES: "I don't feel like sex..." "I could care less..." "I feel bad for my husband..." "It's affecting our relationship..."
2. VAGINAL DRYNESS/DISCOMFORT ISSUES: "...I'm so dry."

---

[1] *For Women Only: A Revolutionary Guide to Overcoming Sexual Dysfunction and Reclaiming Your Sexual Life,* Jennifer Berman, M.D., Laura Berman, PhD and Elizabeth Bunmiller, Henry Holt & Co, 2001.

3. ORGASMIC ISSUES
   a. In women who have no previous history of orgasmic dysfunction: "...I get to the edge, but I can't quite sail off..."
   b. In women who have never been fully orgasmic: "I've faked it at times, but I've never really had an orgasm..."
4. MIDLIFE RELATIONSHIP ISSUES
5. PELVIC SURGERY/TRAUMA
6. PSYCHOLOGICAL CAUSES: BODY IMAGE; SELF ESTEEM; STRESS; DEPRESSION

## 1. DESIRE ISSUES

It has been estimated that 40-45% of pre-menopausal women have some degree of "sexual dysfunction." This figure increases to 85-90% post-menopausally!

I see many women in my office for peri-menopausal / menopausal issues which are affecting their quality of life. We talk about the hot flashes, the insomnia, the memory glitches, mood swings and fatigue. The sexual issues (which are invariably there) usually come at the end (as...an afterthought), in answer to my directed questions, or when I review the "sexual satisfaction" answers on their intake history form. But—usually—it is there.

What do I mean by "desire issues"? Lack of sexual desire (obviously!). Low libido. "Not wanting it." "...I really could care less about sex." (Also see ASEX questionnaire, next page)

More often than not, however, once sexual activities have been initiated (usually by one's mate), they are enjoyable and frequently orgasm follows (although possibly taking longer to achieve). But my patient is rarely the initiator.

The issue is brought up because either she feels that something is "missing," or an edginess has come into the relationship over her lack of sexual desire, or just because she notices the change and feels that she ought to mention it.

It is common for women to have sexual complaints during the peri- and post-menopausal years. The causes are multiple (see below). Unfortunately, many menopausal women are given the message that their drop in libido and diminished sexual sensations are a "...normal part of aging."

They certainly do not have to be! Read on:

**Causes of Diminished Sexual Desire in Women** (These issues can exist singly or in various combinations)

1. "Life disruption."

It's hard to feel sexy if you're bleeding all the time. Or you're sleeping terribly, hot flashing, or just feel tired and ornery. As open and sensual as you

# Arizona Sexual Experiences Scale (ASEX)—Female

INSTRUCTIONS: For each item, please indicate your OVERALL level during the PAST WEEK, including TODAY

| 1. How strong is your sex drive? | | | | | |
|---|---|---|---|---|---|
| 1<br>Extremely<br>Strong | 2<br>Very<br>Strong | 3<br>Somewhat<br>Strong | 4<br>Somewhat<br>Weak | 5<br>Very<br>Weak | 6<br>No<br>Sex Drive |

| 2. How easily are you sexually aroused (turned on)? | | | | | |
|---|---|---|---|---|---|
| 1<br>Extremely<br>Easily | 2<br>Very<br>Easily | 3<br>Somewhat<br>Easily | 4<br>Somewhat<br>Difficult | 5<br>Very<br>Difficult | 6<br>Never<br>Aroused |

| 3. How easily does your vagina become moist or wet during sex? | | | | | |
|---|---|---|---|---|---|
| 1<br>Extremely<br>Easily | 2<br>Very<br>Easily | 3<br>Somewhat<br>Easily | 4<br>Somewhat<br>Difficult | 5<br>Very<br>Difficult | 6<br>Never |

| 4. How easily can you reach an orgasm? | | | | | |
|---|---|---|---|---|---|
| 1<br>Extremely<br>Easily | 2<br>Very<br>Easily | 3<br>Somewhat<br>Easily | 4<br>Somewhat<br>Difficult | 5<br>Very<br>Difficult | 6<br>Never Reach<br>Orgasm |

| 5. Are your orgasms satisfying? | | | | | |
|---|---|---|---|---|---|
| 1<br>Extremely<br>Satisfying | 2<br>Very<br>Satisfying | 3<br>Somewhat<br>Satisfying | 4<br>Somewhat<br>Unsatisfying | 5<br>Very<br>Unsatisfying | 6<br>Can't Reach<br>Orgasm |

**TOTAL**

HOW TO SCORE:
The following are highly correlated with the presence of clinician-diagnosed sexual dysfunction:

- A total ASEX score of 19 or greater; **or**
- Any one item with an individual score of 5 or greater; **or**
- Any three items with individual scores of 4 or greater

may be (might have been), many women get shy and less open if they feel bloated or fat.

2.   Partnership Issues.

Many things fall under this heading. Marital stresses, financial stresses, "staleness," partner's difficulty in getting or maintaining his erection.

3.   Hormonal Issues

This can be either estrogen or testosterone-related (or both). If estrogen is low, or bouncing around, the resulting symptoms are not terribly conducive to sensuality and sexual desire.

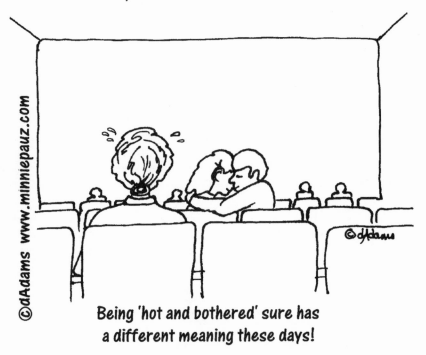

**Being 'hot and bothered' sure has a different meaning these days!**

The very same ovaries that secrete estrogens secrete testosterone as well. Just as all men secrete some estrogen from their testes (their feminine side??), women secrete more than a small amount of androgens: testosterone from their ovaries and DHEA and androstenedione from their adrenal glands. The latter hormones are broken down to testosterone, dihydrotestosterone and estradiol.

Well before your ovaries begin their "swansong," testosterone output begins to wane, slowly but surely (as opposed to the abrupt disruption of estrogen levels accompanying peri-menopause and menopause).

Compounding this lowered testosterone output is the fact that many women "of this age" are put on oral estrogens, or oral contraceptive by their doctors pills for symptoms relief and/or cycle regulation.

By now you know that oral estrogens may increase a blood protein called Sex Hormone Binding Globulin, which decreases by up to 300% the amount of free circulating testosterone, further diminishing testosterone levels (frequently with resultant adverse effects on libido—not exactly what you need!!).

DHEA in the body is metabolized to dihydrotestosterone and estradiol, and has tissue-specific androgen effects of better bone formation, increased sebaceous gland stimulation, mammary gland inhibition and increased muscle mass. It also has estrogenic effects of strengthening vaginal tissue and diminishing insulin resistance (helping prevent diabetes). It does not affect the endometrium.

Beneficial effects of androgens (testosterone, dihydrotestosterone and DHEA) include increased bone mineral density, helping estrogen to diminish hot flashes, and improving libido and sexual satisfaction. Somewhat of a down side in some women is the increased sebum secretion (pimples) and oiliness of skin.

4. Medical and Medication Issues

Of course, if you have another medical condition causing illness, disability, fatigue, etc., this can certainly affect your sexual feelings and response. The most common conditions here are depression, hypertension, diabetes, heart disease and cancer.

Likewise, certain medications used to treat these conditions are a double-edged sword and can diminish sexual desire.

Frequently implicated here are anti-depressant medications (the "tri cyclics") including Elavil®, Anafranil®, Sinequan®, etc.; SSRIs, such as Prozac®, Zoloft®, Paxil®, etc.; and antihypertensive agents (Inderal®, Lopressor®, Corgard®, Tenormin®, Adalat®, Procardia®, Cardiazem®, Calan®, etc., etc.).

Other drugs that can adversely affect sexual response include sedatives (Xanax®, Valium®), certain anticonvulsants and antipsychotic medications, ulcer drugs (Tagamet®) and sometimes birth control pills. If diminishing sexual desire is part of your problem and you are taking these classes of medications, check with your physician about alternatives.

**Therapy for diminished sexual desire**

Just talking about it and the fact that it is an issue is a start!

The first thing to do is accurately identify exactly what is going on. Is it desire ("libido") alone that is at issue, or are there other factors involved (see ASEX questionnaire and understand the other problems of inadequate vaginal lubrication, pain and orgasmic "dysfunction" discussed later in this chapter).

Therapy for "low libido" usually follows one or more of four separate pathways:

1.  Easing peri-menopausal / menopausal symptoms and relieving insomnia.

This should be your first line of therapy. If you are feeling crappy, flash flushing all over the place and sleeping poorly, mad, passionate, sweaty love-making (or <u>any</u> love-making) may not be the first item on your agenda.

Get your hot flashes/night sweats/mood alterations and insomnia under control. (See earlier chapters)

2.  Relieving your vaginal dryness/burning.

Likewise, if you are dry and "it hurts" you're not going to feel like doing it! (Hello...!) There goes desire!

For help with vaginal dryness conditions, see pages 106-107 a little later in this chapter.

3.  TESTOSTERONE

There is a plethora of information from numerous sources that "androgen deficiency" (usually meaning low testosterone) causes problems in women.

In contrast to the acute fall of circulating estrogens at time of menopause, the decline in testosterone output from the ovaries as well as other androgens from the adrenal glands start in the decade leading up to menopause and parallel increasing age. Testosterone goes down before estrogen, steadily and slowly falling, while estrogen usually "spits and sputters" before abruptly declining.

Women may experience symptoms of androgen deficiency in their "late reproductive years" as early as their mid-to-late 30s and beyond. Androgen deficiency symptoms develop insidiously and most women fail to recognize that their symptoms have a biological basis. These include depression, diminished motivation and persistent fatigue, in addition to low libido.

There is no agreed-upon definition of androgen deficiency in women, nor is there any clear-cut laboratory parameter (blood or saliva) at which one can say "Oh, she's low," or conversely, "She's got enough testosterone." So, finding a saliva testosterone level of, say, 22 (at a lab where the "normal range," is 17-57, means little. Maybe this woman's "normal" pre-menopausal levels have always been in the 20s. But maybe they've been in the 40s or 50s, so for <u>her</u> this level is indicative of deficiency.

Treatment parameters, therefore, are based not so much on laboratory test results as on clinical symptoms.

Is your libido low? Self-assertiveness and confidence waning? Loss of energy, diminished sense of well being and vitality? It makes <u>all the sense in the world</u>, then, to try testosterone (and possibly DHEA) supplementation.

There is nothing wrong with getting a testosterone level test (I prefer salivary over blood, as I feel it more accurately reflects tissue level, but it's not an argument I'd put big money on; I frequently get both). If the level is in the mid-high range of normal, I'd repeat it. If it still was "more than fine," I'd consider other causes of this woman's symptoms prior to trying testosterone.

But if the levels are low or in the low end of mid range I'd certainly recommend testosterone supplementation, following testosterone levels periodically to guide increases in dosage and prevent over-treatment.

Gonadal hormones are psychoactive and affect serotonin metabolism (Remember our old friend serotonin of the "feel good" and antidepression fame?) As a generalization, when you add testosterone, then sexual pleasure, orgasm, desire, satisfaction, frequency and relevancy all improve. Adding testosterone to estrogen therapy frequently leads to increased desire and arousal and frequency of sexual activity.

How does testosterone work in your body? What does it do? How does it exert its effect? How is it administered?

Although one of testosterone's metabolic byproducts is estrogen, it is the "stops along the way" that make the difference.

Testosterone (and other androgens) are precursor hormones for some of women's estrogen production, not only in the ovaries but in other tissues as well. Testosterone significantly inhibits bone loss in women, as well as improving brain function, not directly as testosterone, but by its metabolite (or break-down product), estrogen!

How about that!!

This may explain the gender discrepancy in the development of osteoporosis and dementia, which occur much later in life in men than in women, since men maintain adequate circulating testosterone levels for the "non gonadal" production of estrogen in bone and brain well into their later years.

It's a complex metabolic pathway. The ovaries produce estrogen and testosterone and the potent androgen DHEA-sulfate. The adrenals contribute DHEA and androstenedione. Approximately half of circulating testosterone is produced by conversion of DHEA and androstenedione to testosterone. Testosterone is then metabolized to the potent androgen dihydrotestosterone or to estrogen at various sites in the body.

Talk about incestuous relationships! The bottom line is that in replacing estrogen only, a hugely important metabolic factor is being ignored.

Another confounding factor is a blood protein known as "Sex Hormone Binding Globulin," or SHBG, which further serves to regulate testosterone metabolism. The higher the SHBG, the lower the testosterone and vice versa. Therefore stay away from oral estrogens if your libido's gone south!

What are the consequences of low testosterone in women? Testosterone deficiency has been linked to depression, sexual disinterest, and persistent fatigue.

If you are on oral estrogens and suffer from these symptoms, the first order of business is to switch to a transdermal form of administration. Additionally, your physician should consider testosterone replacement if your fatigue, sexual disinterest and/or flatness of mood persists.

## METHODS OF TESTOSTERONE REPLACEMENT:

There are many methods of replacing testosterone. They may be classified as old, new, and "to come."

OLD (just because it's old doesn't mean it's not effective...)

With one exception, all commercial-pharmacy-available methods of testosterone supplementation are manufactured for men, and dosages must be adjusted. That exception is the combined oral estrogen and testosterone pill known as Estratest® and Estratest-HS® (half strength).

Methyltestosterone (or "Android®") used to come in 10 mg tablets, which could be quartered, giving a reasonably effective female dose of 2.5 mg. Unfortunately, the company has, as of this writing, stopped making methyltestosterone in tablets; breaking down the 10 mg capsules presently available and re-inserting ⅕-¼ into small gel caps is possible, but arduous!

Fluoxymesterone (or "Halotestin®") comes in 5 and 10 mg tablets; a good woman's dose is 1-2 mg per day.

Testosterone patches are available but in dosages generally too high for women's use.

(RELATIVELY) NEW:

Many mid-sized towns and most larger cities have a compounding pharmacy, a place where the pharmacist mixes or "compounds" medications to your exact specifications, with both the dose, compound, and delivery system fashioned to work for you. Both estrogens, DHEA, pregnenolone, progesterone, and, of course, testosterone, can be compounded into both oral and (preferably) transdermal forms in lotions, creams, gels, or troches ("lozenges"). A skilled nurse practitioner or physician savvy in compounding and transdermal application can help you with this (see Chapter 20).

Although oral micronized testosterone (a bioidentical) 1-3 mg and compounded methyltestosterone (a synthetic) 1-3 mg are fine, my favorite way of supplementing testosterone is via a lotion, starting at a concentration of 10 mg per cc. Doses vary, but I usually start with approximately ½ cc (5 mg) per day, going after 1-2 weeks to 0.2-0.3 cc (2-3 mg) per day. This may be used any time of day; bedtime may work best.

Where do you apply the cream/lotion? On soft skin (inner aspects of upper arms, inner thighs, labia). Certainly, if testosterone is being used to improve libido, applying cream to the labia (inner lips and clitoral area) may get you more..."involved."

You don't have to be alone in this application! Your mate can certainly help (this may lead to "bigger and better things"—who knows?). In fact, you can put a bit onto your sweetie's penis (no harm done) and kid him about its anticipated effects... (there certainly are advantages using locally applied testosterone and sometimes estrogen as well to the clitoris/vulva. But make sure your clinician watches testosterone levels periodically as absorption is excellent from these areas).

If you appear to be resistant to testosterone therapy, ask your doc to measure both free and total testosterone and perhaps also SHBG (especially if you're on oral estrogens).

TO COME:

On the horizon from Proctor and Gamble (that venerable bastion of home hygiene aids) are testosterone patches for women, available in 3 dosage strengths and changed once-twice per week.

Also possible: testosterone spray (in alcohol base). (Hey—a quick breath spray in your mouth and a little testosterone spray "down there" and you're all ready. What an image!)

4.  SELF AWARENESS

Testosterone levels notwithstanding, there's always room for work in this area. So often "libido depletion" (both women and men) stems from boredom, sameness, body image uncertainties, and a limited repertoire of sexual ideas.

Here's a wonderful and relatively easy treatment modality that you can try at home. I call it a "four step method to sexual rejuvenation," but actually it is no more than the "PLISSIT" model first suggested by Kaplan, and Hartman and Fithian, among others. PLISSIT is an acronym for Permission, Limited Information, Simple Suggestions, and (if needed) Intensive Therapy. It works by self-awareness and desensitization. You need a month or three and the full cooperation of your sexual partner. You also need to put aside adequate time, which will be well-rewarded later.

Here's the program, in outline form:

1.  Secure the cooperation of your partner, eliciting his agreement to abstain from all mutual sexual activities until you "invite him in" (usually in several weeks) and then abstain from penile intercourse until you are ready (another few weeks). Of course, make it clear that your sweetie may engage in "self pleasuring," provided no personal or religious proscription precludes this.

2.  Set aside approximately 30 minutes at least twice a week (3-4 times are much preferred) to learn all about yourself and your body. About its likes and dislikes, sensitivities, soft spots and erotic areas. The door to your bedroom or bathroom is locked! No one is allowed to disturb you!

You may lie naked in bed or better yet is a warm water tub. Lights dim. (Candles are nice.) Soft music, if you want. Maybe a glass of wine. You get the picture.

Explore yourself, looking and gently touching as you go. What feels good to touch? Exactly where? Exactly how? Hard? Soft? Lightly stroked? Vigorously massaged? Although this has to do with self-exploration and discovery, if something feels real good and you wish to linger, you may.

This is not a one-time affair. Continue for as many sessions as it takes (most women say 5-10 times (some more, some less) to understand the ins and outs of your body. Its contours and nooks and crannies. Most importantly, what feels good and what does not. What you like to touch/have touched, to look at/have looked at, to talk about/have talked about, as well as what you do not like, so that you can later clearly instruct your partner.

2a. Next, the same thing, but linger awhile if it feels good. Play, enjoy and experience orgasm if...it happens.

3.   When you are ready, invite your husband/partner in (bed or tub). Show him what you like. What feels good. How and what you like to be talked to/talk about. And ask him for the same information. One rule must be established beforehand: no penile intercourse. Self and mutual pleasuring is fine. Orgasm is fine. But no penetration.

4.   When you are ready, invite your lover to enter you—or better, you put him inside. For now, you control this. You call the shots.

5.   Whenever you are ready..."you are on your own."

Addendum: Don't forget the power of fantasy, of erotica. In sex, as long as it hurts no one and there is mutual agreement, everything is fair game. Visual fantasies, spoken fantasies (even of things you never dream of doing in reality), implements of pleasure and erotic literature are all wonderful. Think about these additions yourself and discuss them with your mate. The erotica section of your local bookstore, adult bookstore and online sources are great places to browse (see Chapter 20). For sensual erotic literature, practically any book written or edited by Lonnie Barbach is great.

Obviously, this program requires some time and of course the full cooperation of your partner. And frequently, short, selective "brush up sessions" are helpful. But, the rewards are enormous.

## 2.   VAGINAL DRYNESS/DISCOMFORT ISSUES

This is obvious. If you feel dry and scratchy, sex can feel like sandpapering a sore.

A woman's "sex skin" (vulva, vagina and perineum) is most sensitive to declining levels of both estrogen and testosterone. Along with changing menstrual patterns, hot flashes and fatigue, vaginal dryness is one of the classic hassles of (peri-) menopause.

Not infrequently, diminished blood supply to the vulva and/or scarification resulting from pelvic surgery can cause discomfort and dryness and interfere with orgasm (see "orgasmic issues" for further discussion of this).

Therapy:

Although it doesn't necessarily indicate arousal, a little lubrication goes a long way!

A course of topical estrogens helps. This can include an estrogen vaginal cream, a foaming estradiol vaginal insert tablet (Vagifem®)—less messy than cream—or Estring®, a small ring-shaped vaginal pessary imbedded with estrogen. One of these will usually in relatively short order supply your vagina with enough local hormonal support to feel less "rough" and better lubricated. (Frequently it's probably a good idea to use vaginal estrogens even if you begin to take oral or transdermal estrogen therapy, as it frequently takes many months for these systemic therapies to fully affect the vagina.

In the meantime, however, local lubrication may be invaluable.

There are two choices (oil based or water based) and each has advantages and disadvantages. Oil based lubricants (baby oil, light olive oil, light massage oil, etc.) can be wonderfully sensual. Each of you pour a little into your hands, rub them together to warm the oil, and ...play. The oil can be mutually applied wherever you wish, especially to those parts where "friction" might be a problem. An added advantage is that some form of light oil is available in most every household.

The down side to oil? It can be a bit messy if you slop it around; oil can break down latex if condoms are your contraceptive method; it can lead to vaginal infection recurrence if you are troubled by easily recurring vaginal infections.

Water based lubricants (Astroglide®, Silky®, etc.) have as their active ingredients glycerol and propylene glycol, which accounts for their "slippery" feel. Water based lubricants are also fun to play with, but can be "colder" than oil and, as opposed to oil, can dry out and get tacky.

A moisturizing agent such as Replens® may be used well prior to sexual activity (or not even associated with sex) to increase vaginal moisture and help with the moment-to-moment feelings of dryness and scratchiness.

## 3.  ORGASMIC ISSUES

Are you aware that only a small percentage (approximately 30%) of women experience orgasm with penile intercourse alone? (So much for "wham bam, thank you ma'am" sex!) This does not mean that only a small percentage of women are orgasmic—only that in a majority of women or couples, other modes (self or mutual manual or oral stimulation, use of a vibrator or dildo, spoken or visual fantasy, etc.) are necessary for a woman to achieve orgasm. Men sometimes have trouble with this (Get over it!) but nothing that a bit of sensitive counseling and discussion can't solve.

That's said, it is not uncommon for previously orgasmic women passing through midlife to have greater difficulty "going over the edge."

The reasons are tied up with many of the things already mentioned and discussed below: peri-menopausal hormonal issues, fatigue, vaginal dryness, discomfort in one's relationship, etc.

Another factor significantly impacting orgasmic ability is the anatomic and physiologic issue of diminished blood supply with aging and pelvic surgery. Just as a man's erection is caused by blood filling up that skin-coated spongy cylinder called a penis, the clitoral and vaginal wall engorgement that precedes orgasmic relief is dependent on good, intact blood and nerve supply, both of which can be affected by aging and/or pelvic surgery.

Women who have never (or extremely rarely) been previously orgasmic have a different issue (although still potentially affected by their midlife passage), as will be discussed when we later look at treatment ideas.

Therapy for "orgasmic issues" (not having or extreme difficulty in achieving an orgasm) differs between women who used to be orgasmic but have lost that ability in the peri-menopause, and women who have never been orgasmic. For the former, frequently the peri-menopausal change of diminished blood supply to the vulva leads to an inadequate road to the "plateau" that precedes orgasmic release. If this is the case (not an arousal issue but an orgasmic issue) in a previously orgasmic woman, two therapeutic approaches (alone or in combination) can work great.

1.  Sildenafil

Sildenafil, better known by its trade name Viagra®, has brought untold millions of dollars to Pfizer and has erected many a penis. It also works in a limited but very successful way for previously orgasmic women who have OK desire, but increasing difficulty in achieving orgasm. The dose is 25-50 mg (as it's so expensive and not covered by most insurance, have your doctor prescribe the 50 mg dose and cut the tablets in half with a pill cutter. If you find that 50 mg is your effective dose, get the 100 mg tablets and cut in half. It works and is much more cost effective). Sildenafil can help also with arousal, lubrication and increased genital sensations if other methods described earlier are inadequate. It is best taken ½-1 hour prior to planned love-making.

Sildenafil helps dilate genital blood vessels resulting in subsequent clitoral, vulvar and vaginal erectile tissue engorgement.

Based on sildenafil's mechanism of action, post-menopausal women with vascular disease, hypertension, and diabetes who have normal libido and hormones may also be ideal candidates for therapy.

Sildenafil is specifically good in arousal and orgasmic difficulties, as distinguished from desire disorders.

2. Eros CSD

Spelled out: Eros Clitoral Stimulation Device. This is a nifty little unit (by prescription only) which gently attaches by suction to the clitoris. By regular usage, the gentle suction activity slowly swells your clitoris making it more sensitive and responsive (and used to the stimulation).

For many women it works. Ask your MD or therapist about it, or contact UroMetrics at (877) 774-1442 or http://www.UroMetrics.com for more information. Although covered by some insurances, the cost is pretty steep (around $400). If it works, however, it's a small price to pay.

For women who have pretty much never been orgasmic, therapy follows the "PLISSIT" model outlined previously.

This regimen, best supervised by a therapist, is both a good structure toward increasing sexual desire and the establishment of better orgasmic function (in other words, feeling relaxed enough, excited enough, "out of control enough" to enjoy the power and release of orgasm).

In this approach, one is given permission to be open, to explore, to be candid, to observe, touch and reach into one's body and the body of one's partner. Information regarding anatomy, erogenous zones, response, self and mutual pleasuring (permission enters in here also) is encouraged. Simple suggestions for pleasure-enhancing self and mutual sexual activities are given. Usually, somewhere along the line, orgasm occurs. If not, then the last (intensive therapy) can often chase away the Freudian and other ghosts so that the elusive "big O" can see the light of day.

This regimen takes time and incorporates many of the techniques discussed earlier in Sexual Rejuvenation. It works. But in treating "anorgasmia" it's not necessarily something you'll try alone. A good guide is priceless.

4. **MIDLIFE RELATIONSHIP ISSUES**

Obviously, if you and your partner are fighting or have unresolved issues, you are usually not going to be approaching each other sexually (although it is a great way to "make up"). Life with another person is frequently a struggle and the stresses of midlife add to that struggle.

This is where a good therapist comes in. Psychologists (Ph.D. or Psy.D.), psychiatrists, licensed clinical social workers (LCSWs) and marriage and family therapists (MFCs) all come from somewhat different training backgrounds, with MD psychiatrists being the only ones who can prescribe medications; but all can be effective as counselors. The psychologists, MFCs and social workers are probably better (and have more time and are less expensive) at "talk therapy" and you can have your OB/GYN or primary care physician write prescriptions if necessary. It really comes down to whom you trust, whose insight is helpful for you, and whom you work best with.

Understand: Therapists are people also and each brings her or his own biases and experiences into the therapeutic setting. (Why do you think many went into the field of psychotherapy in the first place?) While you definitely are not looking for a "yes man" (or woman) who simply validates your biases, you must have someone that you—and your mate—respect and trust.

I'll repeat: and your mate!! It's hard to do this in a vacuum.

## 5.  PELVIC SURGERY / TRAUMA

Not necessarily a cause of sexual desire issues, pelvic surgery especially and occasional vaginal area trauma may interfere with blood and nerve supply to the labia (specifically the clitoris) and vagina. This diminished blood supply may lead to inadequate moisture and lubrication and difficulty with vaginal and clitoral engorgement, making orgasm difficult.

Sildenafil (Viagra) can be quite useful here, helping to increase blood supply (and therefore engorgement) of the vulva/vagina/clitoris.

Along the lines of prevention, if you are to have pelvic surgery (hysterectomy, pelvic support surgery) discuss specifically with your surgeon the concept of a "nerve sparing and vascular sparing" procedure. This may include doing a "supracervical hysterectomy" (removing the uterus but leaving the cervix in place) and avoiding as much blood vessel and nerve disruption as possible.

## 6.  PSYCHOLOGICAL CAUSES

Perception of body image, poor self esteem, stress and depression can at any time serve to diminish sexual desire. At midlife certainly, many of these things may be magnified. Your sexuality does not exist in a vacuum and is certainly affected and modified by these issues.

Midlife women frequently suffer from a low level depression known as "dysthymia," noticing themselves not really excited about things and experiencing a diminished *joie de vivre.*

First line therapy for refractory (treatment resistant) dysthymia/ depression consists of SSRIs (Celexa®, Zoloft®, Prozac®, etc.) However, if these agents, while perhaps helping with the depressive symptoms, act to further diminish sexual response, ask your therapist to consider adding buproprion (Wellbutrin-SR®) to the regimen. Other good antidepressants which have less adverse effect on libido are Serzone® and Remeron®. If your psychological pattern is consistent with or if you have been diagnosed with ADHD (attention deficit hyperactivity disorder), and you experience orgasmic difficulties (but your libido is OK), consider trying Concerta® (long-acting ritalin)

If sexual problems remain after assessment for relationship issues and psychological illness, re-establishment of vaginal health and therapy of the central issues of mood, hot flashes, etc. and testosterone therapy, you should probably <u>return</u> to the possibility of your having incompletely treated dysthymia/depression as well as subtle relationship issues. Certainly stress can also play a role (see Chapter 13).

So, you see, sexual desire issues (or so-called "sexual dysfunction"—a phrase I dislike) are certainly multi-factorial at midlife. Simply "throwing a little testosterone on the waters" may be too simplistic an approach (although frequently a good place to start).

If suboptimal sexual functioning is part of your midlife passage, re-read this chapter carefully, think about where you may fit in and explain, describe and perhaps guide your physician and/or therapist to a good resolution.

## CHLOE'S STORY

Chloe Davis' neighbor had recommended me to her. Chloe was 39, but three years earlier, after a period of irregular menses she had stopped altogether and was diagnosed with having "premature ovarian failure" or ... "early menopause." She had been on PremPro®, but stopped it 2 months ago out of worry and because she "didn't like to take them." She was now having serious hot flashes and difficulty sleeping.

I was to discover this much in the first minutes of our interview. She hadn't had much of a previous workup other than a couple of tests for FSH (both were quite elevated; FSH, which stands for follicle stimulating hormone, cause the ovaries to mature an egg); she was started on hormone replacement therapy.

As we progressed in our interview and I asked her if she was sexually active and about her degree of sexual satisfaction, she stated that she had very little desire and that this was a thorn between her and her husband. I asked her to fill out an ASEX questionnaire, which is reproduced below.

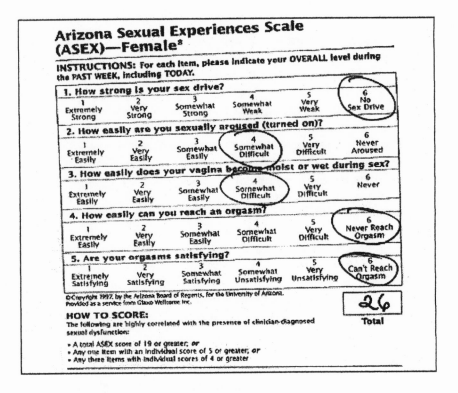

After I'd run a few tests, to confirm that Chloe's FSH was still elevated and her thyroid was normal, and to rule out an "autoimmune" cause for her situation, we negotiated an HRT regimen that worked for her. Because of her sexual desire situation and other reasons, we decided on an estradiol patch (we both liked the idea of the small size of the Vivelle-Dot®) and a low dose of NET (which was covered by her insurance). She wanted to start low on the HRT, so I helped her hot flash and insomnia problems for a few weeks with Effexor® and occasionally Ambien® to help with her sleep. She did not feel the need to take these "crutches," as she called them (but initially a welcome crutch) after 3 weeks.

We'd spoken briefly at our first visit about her sexual situation and elected to add in a dose of transdermal testosterone lotion both for libido reasons and to increase the effectiveness of the low dose transdermal estrogen therapy. We put her lack of orgasms off for later, but promised each other that we'd return to it in awhile.

In view of the ovarian failure, I felt it was warranted to start testosterone even before I received the results of Chloe's first salivary testosterone level, which I got anyway for a baseline. I was not surprised when it came back quite low at 13.9 (17-52 was normal for this lab).

Also, as Chloe was relatively high risk because of her "early menopause," I advised at least a peripheral (if not central) bone density measurement.

At her 10-day follow up, she had her annual exam and Pap and I performed a brief ultrasound of her ovaries and confirmed that she had obtained and was doing OK on her new meds.

Chloe then returned one month after her first visits. She was off the "psychoactives" and reported that her hot flashes were "90% better" and she was sleeping well. She also had noted a definitive increase in her energy and a modest improvement in sexual desire.

I asked her if she still wanted to work on her orgasmic situation and she replied in the affirmative. Although her premature ovarian failure could have altered blood supply to her vulva, in which case sildenafil might be helpful, arousal was only part of the issue. She had never had an orgasm with penile or other stimulation. Although she had "awoken hot and bothered" a couple of times in her youth, she didn't masturbate, so couldn't speak to being orgasmic with self-pleasuring.

I outlined my usual therapeutic approach and encouraged her to invite her husband to our next session. "He's very much a part of this," I said. "And you'll need his cooperation and encouragement. He doesn't have to come to all of the sessions, but of course he's invited."

"I don't think he'll want to come," Chloe replied. "Steve's not too keen on therapy or coming to a gynecologist—he told me just to do whatever I needed to."

As predicted, Steve didn't accompany Chloe to her next visit one week later, at which time I inquired deeply into Chloe's childhood and her parental and religious background; to gain exposure to her parents' sexuality and attitudes, and to her earlier sexual experiences, as well as to her lovemaking pattern with Steve.

"I was raised in an average suburban household with 2 older brothers. I am Presbyterian by heritage and my parents attended church regularly, but I go only occasionally."

She couldn't recollect any rigidity or proscriptions regarding sex, although it was something that wasn't discussed one way or the other in her household. She had once walked in on her parents during their lovemaking when she was a teenager; she described them as being more embarrassed than she.

Her sexual experiences, both earlier ("I dated a lot") and with her husband were pretty much along the lines of "stick it in and get it on." She was not really embarrassed about masturbation, she just "really hadn't done it."

I once again outlined the therapeutic mode. She would start out at least 2 but hopefully 3-4 times a week with simple looking and touching self-discovery in a relaxed setting, preferably the tub in warm water, maybe with some bath salts. "All you're to do is look at, touch, and if you want, talk about each part of your body. Your hair to your toes. No negative comments.. No good or bad. You have my permission to explore and to note what feels good (and what doesn't). If you want to linger and/or enjoy any particular area, you may. For example, you may discover that, while you like to be caressed lightly on the tips of your nipples and on the soft skin on the under surface of your breasts, that you are uncomfortable and ticklish when your nipples and areola are pulled. Notice stuff like that," I told her.

"During this phase, which may last a couple of weeks, maybe a month, and during the next phase, you are not to have intercourse, you know. Is Steve OK with that? This is a no-pressure, self-discovery time to use to (re)acquaint yourself with your body. I want to touch base with you—briefly or at length—by phone or here during this time to see how you're faring."

I again encouraged her husband to be a more direct part of the plan, but Chloe said she'd discussed it with him (including the abstinence) after our last visit and that he was "on board." I agreed to continue, but left the door open for more of his active participation.

Since she hadn't called, I contacted Chloe a week later. She admitted she'd only explored once since our visit. She felt awkward. "That's all right," I encouraged. "It's usually that way at first, but I really <u>do</u> want you to do this at least 3 times a week." Chloe asked if exploring in her bed was OK, as the tub "felt funny." I said OK and she certainly could return to the tub, if she wanted.

Two weeks later, Chloe returned. She was doing fine on the HRT. A repeat salivary testosterone was now 25.5 (in the lower part of the normal range) and I asked her to increase her nightly dose by about 25%. "You know," she told me, "for the first couple of times, I wasn't at all sure about this. But I've continued and actually explored four times last week, and you know, I'm not so shy and actually like it."

Steve was being real good but he was definitely hinting that he'd "sure like to be part of her discoveries." We talked about "fiddling around" with a vibrator and she'd admitted that she'd already ordered one ("I won't dare tell you the shape") from the Good Vibrations website, which she'd found on the Resource Sheet I'd given her.

To make a not-too-long story shorter, Chloe discovered that, where she was able to enjoy and "get to the edge" with manual stimulation (which Steve helped with when she "invited him in" a week later, still with the ban on intercourse), she still wasn't quite orgasmic. The arrival of the vibrator, however, changed all that and she "now knew what it felt like."

Chloe and Steve are making love, including intercourse, now, and although she hasn't yet experienced a climax with Steve's penis, she (and Steve!) feel quite comfortable using the vibrator.

"My desire is no problem now (her last salivary testosterone came back at 44—normal), and I even attacked Steve last week—was he surprised!"

*One has two duties: to be worried and not to be worried.*
—E.M. Forster

# CHAPTER NINE

## HORMONES AND BREAST CANCER
(Not as scary as you thought)

I'm going to try to make this a short chapter. Not because this isn't an important topic. Not because most women aren't fearful of breast cancer. Not because I'm sure <u>everyone</u> reading this book has had a friend, neighbor, or relative who has had breast cancer, or knows someone who has.

Genetics aside, the greatest risks to a woman are her own ovaries. The estrogens they secrete are of far greater potency than even high dose estrogen supplementation. That is why early menarche, late menopause, childlessness, or late first child are all positive risk factors for breast cancer: they all expose the breasts to longer term and/or higher levels of estrogen. The increased risk produced by estrogen therapy is secondary to increasing, for long periods of time beyond that naturally expected for a given individual, an estrogen-rich milieu.. Conversely, anything which can be expected to <u>decrease</u> estrogen levels over a woman's lifetime (late menarche, early menopause, many children, especially with nursing over 6 months, thus diminishing estrogen levels) can be considered protective.

An example may be helpful: Identical twin sisters are 35 years old and both have 2 children and nursed them. Because of a life-threatening pelvic infection, one twin has had a total hysterectomy with removal of her ovaries and begins, at age 35, mid-dose estrogen replacement therapy (ERT), let's say Premarin® 1.25 mg, tapering down to low dose ERT (let's say Premarin® 0.625 mg) at age 50. The twins are now both 55 years old and the other twin has just gone through menopause. "Twin A" has been on ERT for 20 years; "Twin B" has had no hormone supplementation other than her own ovarian cycling. Which twin is at greater risk for breast cancer?

It may surprise you to know that it is Twin B who is at higher risk because her total estrogen exposure (with her ovaries) has been much higher over this 20-year period than that given in the form of estrogen supplementation to her sister.

It has to do with hormone levels and individual breast sensitivity toward developing breast cancer, and random mutations. An obese woman has a greater overall risk of breast cancer. Fat is broken down into estrogen-like substances; there may be dietary factors as well. A lean woman, one with low body mass index (BMI), because of her lower level of circulating estrogens than her more substantial sister, has lesser risk of breast cancer. However, when a lean woman takes long term HRT, her risk of getting breast cancer is higher than therapy bestows on larger women because she is taking more estrogen per pound of body weight, thus exposing her breasts to a higher estrogen environment.

Breast cancer, in most cases, arises spontaneously by a chance sequence of abnormal mutations and is influenced by the body's production of enzymes and other factors which regulate cell growth. Hormones can act on cancer cells by increasing or decreasing DNA replication, thus affecting the rate of cell division. Available data suggest that estrogen level is a factor in many breast cancers.

Denser breast tissue (more glandular tissue) is a subtle risk factor; these women tend to have more breast biopsies as well because it is more difficult to identify benign vs. cancerous tissue in denser breasts.

How does all this relate to the individual's decision whether or not to use HRT? What are the different risk/benefit ratios in the "low risk" woman, the "high risk" woman or a woman with previous history of breast cancer or "pre-cancer" on a recent biopsy?

A recent meta-analysis (translation: grand review of many studies) of more than 750,000 women, as well as several new studies all show no evidence of increased risk of breast cancer in women taking low dose, short-term estrogen supplementation. The key is "short term," and "low dose."

What is meant by "short term"?? Probably anything less than 4-5 years; certainly less than 2-3 years.

So, re-visit the chapters on HRT and alternatives. There's no need to suffer unnecessarily. Herbs and botanicals may do it. But also helpful might be for you to take control of your peri-menopause by eating naturally and well and exercising regularly. Also possibly starting a low dose bioidentical estrogen supplementation.

This does not have to be forever! After symptoms are well controlled, say, for a year, use the next 1-2 years to slowly and imperceptibly taper down or off altogether.

What about a woman with past history or a very recent breast cancer diagnosis with adjunct chemo or x-ray therapy that has hastened the menopausal process—and now she's suffering mightily?

It may surprise you to know the results of several recent studies of breast cancer survivors and other women recently treated for breast cancer. The death rate from breast cancer for the group of women who took HRT for approximately 2 years or less to "smooth out" their transition was actually less than the group who did not take estrogens (2-3 times less, even when corrected for other factors which might falsely increase survival in the estrogen-treated group). This doesn't mean I can tell you as a breast cancer survivor, to be unequivocally comfortable with estrogen therapy. If, each time you put on the patch or take the pill you're scared to death, of course you don't want to be taking estrogens (think of the psychic damage you're doing to your immune system if you have negative feelings each time you "dose up").

So, if you're high risk or a breast cancer survivor and are not comfortable with systemic estrogens, what do you do?

1. Vaginal dryness: Use a topically applied product in the vagina, with little estrogen absorption. The Estring® (vaginal estradiol ring, good for 3 months) releases the least amount of estradiol daily. It's OK to use a vaginal estrogen cream, but use at ¼ the recommended doses (¼ applicator full every other night, after 2-3 weeks of full nightly doses).

2. Hot flashes, mood changes, etc.: Best you can do (besides avoiding the "triggers" described previously) is botanicals (isoflavones, black cohosh, perhaps chasteberry, etc.—see Chapter 7) plus 800 mg vitamin E per day and Effexor® or some other SSRI (serotonin enhancers, or "feel good" medication). Also, high dose progestin therapy such as Megace® or Provera® or ½ tsp. of 3-5% Progesterone cream, or a compounded 50-100 mg dose nightly can bring hot flash relief.

But, as I noted earlier, the long-held belief that women at high risk for breast cancer cannot or should not take replacement hormone therapy or estrogen supplementation is wrong. (Stated another way: It seems that women who use hormonal supplementation after breast cancer are not at increased risk for recurrence or death.) THE KEY IS (regardless of dose), SHORT TIME. (I usually recommend for 2 years or less; some data indicate up to 5 years is safe, some only 18 months.) The role of dosage of hormone replacement/supplementation and the exact compounds or delivery systems is unclear. Are bioidenticals (e.g., estradiol, estriol) any more or less risky than synthetics (e.g., conjugated estrogens, ethinyl estradiol)? Are transdermals any more or less safe than pills? Common sense (and some data) indicate that lower doses are safer, but even this is not for sure. It will be years (at least 5-10) before we have more definitive answers to these questions. Understand also: the increased incidence of breast cancer in women who have taken long term (5 or more years) post-menopausal HRT is actually less than that associated with post-menopausal obesity or alcohol consumption in excess of 1 drink per day.

My recommendation: take control of your passage, whether that is by nutrition, supplements, botanicals or hormones. If you elect HRT, after your symptoms are well controlled (for at least 6-12 months), start a very slow, imperceptible taper-down to zero (or super low dose, if you wish) over a period of the next 1-2 years.

If not using estrogens, check your bone density periodically (I'd recommend a peripheral-heel-screen every 2 years; if it's OK, fine; if decreased, follow up with a central bone density exam (e.g., DEXA).

Also interesting: Women who develop breast cancer while taking post-menopausal HRT have a reduced risk of dying from breast cancer! This is because of two factors: increased surveillance and early detection, and acceleration of pre-existing tumor growth so that tumors appear at a less virulent and aggressive stage.

One key to the whole question of the relationship of estrogens to breast cancer is a little item known as the "estrogen receptor." These are like little "locks" in the tissue. Breast tissue, bone tissue, brain tissue, skin, etc., etc. Different substances (i.e., estrogens and the group of "anti-estrogens," SERMs) can attach or "key into" these locks and by so doing elicit certain effects, including cancer causality and prevention, prevention of bone loss, effect on skin elasticity, vaginal lubrication, etc., etc.

## THE PLACE OF SERMS IN HRT AND EFFECTS ON BREAST CANCER

Selective Estrogen Receptor Modulators are compounds synthesized to "look like estrogens" (and therefore "fill" the estrogen receptor slots in some tissues-bone and breast especially), but actually act like anti-estrogens (have effects opposite to those of estrogens) in breast tissue. SERMS are not estrogens.

SERMs have an unequivocal place in both therapy and prevention of breast cancer.

Tamoxifen (Nolvadex®) is frequently used as chemotherapy for 3-5 years after conservative surgery (e.g., lumpectomy, occasionally mastectomy) for tumors with positive estrogen receptors. The theory is that the tamoxifen fills the estrogen receptor sites in breast and peripheral tissue, minimizing risk of cancer recurrence or of a new cancer.

Ask your PCP or GYN to run a "Gail Model" on you. This is a short, easy-to-do computer statistical analysis that can determine your individual relative risk for developing breast cancer. It takes into account your current age, number of first degree relatives with breast cancer, age at menarche, number of children and if you nursed, your age at your first birth, and the number of breast biopsies that you've had (and whether any showed atypia).

This analysis helps identify women who are at risk, for increased surveillance and medical preventive measures, and to reassure some women who had previously overestimated their risk of breast cancer.

Two important uses of SERMs:

1. If your GAIL Model is equal to or over 2 (some say 1.7), meaning that you have a two times relative risk of getting breast cancer, you may want to take a SERM (tamoxifen, possibly raloxifene) to lower that cumulative risk.

2. Given the protective effect of SERMs (raloxifene or Evista® and the soon-to-be-available tibolone—see Chapter 18) on breast cancer and bone density, these agents may become the preferred choices for long-term therapy in post-menopausal women who benefit from HRT.

## SEXUALITY AFTER BREAST CANCER

Breast cancer frequently affects sexual function, response, and couples' relationships, involving both psychological and biological factors.

Although 70-80% of breast cancer survivors have a positive overall psychological adjustment and quality of life, this is not true for sexual functioning and satisfaction.

What can you do and how can you work with your practitioner? You should look at symptom areas: libido, sexual arousal, orgasm, satisfaction, relationship issues and HRT (as discussed in Chapter 8).

Testosterone may be helpful here, as may sildenafil (Viagra®). Improving vaginal lubrication is a must and has been previously discussed. Individual and couples psychotherapy is extremely helpful in maintaining a sexual relationship and improving satisfaction. A period of re-exploration of your possibly-changed body, as well as re-establishing and re-discovering your sensuality is important. As mentioned in Chapter 8, exploration of erotica and sexual fantasy and discussion with your mate is very helpful.

## SUMMARY

1. What can you do to diminish your risk of breast cancer, considering that you can't alter your genetics and, so far as I'm aware, there is no cosmic way of altering random cell mutations?

    Diet: Cut down on animal fats; increase fresh fruits, veggies, beans, grains, fish, etc.

    Lifestyle: Increase exercise and watch caloric intake. Obesity increases breast cancer risk. Keep alcohol consumption to a minimum (the best beverage would be wine, preferably red, or beer; not over 1 per day). Limit or quit smoking.

Medications: Consider a SERM premenopausally if at increased risk for breast cancer. Consider a SERM post-menopausally, especially if prevention of bone loss is additionally important.

2. What can you do to increase your odds of early detection?

Self-exam: I suggest practically every day a quick check in the shower to familiarize yourself with your breast consistency. Just as you know subconsciously what the engine of your car sounds like, you should know what your breasts feel like so that you will notice subtle changes and point them out to your health care practitioner. Additionally good is a formal and careful manual and visual check every 1-2 months.

Mammography: Definitely improves early detection. I'd recommend every 2-3 years after age 40 and every 1-2 years after age 50 in low risk women; possibly every 2 years starting at age 35 and yearly after age 40 in high risk women. Ask your practitioner for his/her advice.

New Methodology: Ductal lavage, thermography, etc., may be appropriate for the very high risk woman. See Chapter 18 for details.

3. General rules on estrogen supplementation: Low dose and short duration appears quite safe to deal with disconcerting peri-menopausal symptoms even in the high risk woman and cancer survivors. What else is there to say?

4. What about herbs and botanicals: No risk, except greatly increasing your isoflavones (in excess of 150 mg per day) appears to increase breast cancer risk.

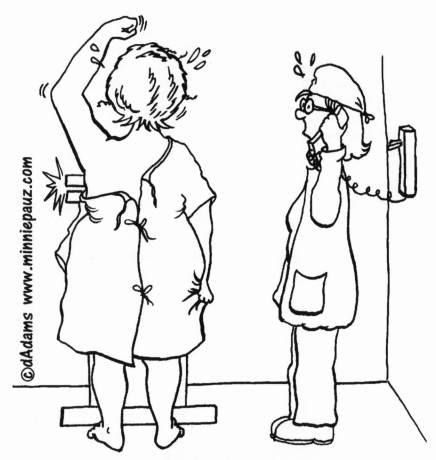

**Marge, come quick! I think I've won the contest for the highest compression!!**

## SHIRLEY'S STORY

Shirley Baletti came right to the point: "I'm too darned dry," she complained. "It burns and it scratches."

Shirley had recently celebrated her 61st birthday by "getting involved," was the way she had put it. "Leon is such a sweetie. He's so patient. He likes to do things with his lips, see...but we haven't been able to have intercourse because I'm so tender. I heard you speak at that seminar and I thought you might be able to help."

As we progressed, I discovered that Shirley had been on Tamoxifen® as a preventive for 2½ years after a lumpectomy for Stage 1a1 carcinoma of her left breast. Prior to her diagnosis, she had been on HRT ("PremPro®") for 10 years. She was angry and felt sure the estrogens were responsible for her tumor which, she informed me, "had positive estrogen receptors."

She was very active, hiking and skiing every chance she got. The hot flashes and moodiness that followed her switch from HRT to Tamoxifen®, which "pushed me in the opposite direction" had been difficult, and only very slightly tempered by (in order) soy isoflavones, Estrovan®, vitamin E, Effexor® and even high doses of DepoProvera®. Although the hot flashes had tempered significantly on the DepoProvera®, she hadn't liked the fluid retention and was concerned by new data which suggested that long-term DepoProvera® may have an adverse effect on bone density.

"Osteoporosis runs in my family, and when I had a DEXA 10 years ago, my bone density was a little low," she told me.

Shirley was a professor of English at the university in the city where I practice, and was a no-nonsense person. After her exam, which showed no evidence of any vulvar dystrophies (benign irregularities around the vaginal entrance) which might account for her symptoms, and a brief ultrasound of the uterus to check for uterine microglandular hyperplasia which frequently accompanies tamoxifen therapy, we discussed her situation.

"Now that the DepoProvera® is wearing off, the hot flashes are returning and I'm still not sleeping well."

Her first item of business, though, was vaginal functioning. I described an Estring®, and she liked the idea. I also suggested adding in ¼ applicator-full of estradiol cream for the first two weeks, massaged into her perineum and placed in the vagina, to "better prepare things" prior to trying love-making. We also discussed lubrication and she definitely was with the program when I intimated the joys of massage oil...

As our hour together wound down, Shirley brought up some other minor symptoms and asked about therapeutic options. I armed her with several articles speaking to hormone and alternative therapy in breast cancer survivors, and we made a 3-week follow-up appointment.

At her return, after we'd settled into my office, Shirley gave me a pixie-like grin and informed me that "it's working." Although a tad tender and relatively short-lived, I learned that "Leon is as good with his wand as he is with his tongue."

We were delighted.

She still, however, wasn't sleeping well and her hot flashes were a bother.

"It's unusual," I told her, "that these symptoms are still a problem at your age and after this long a time on the Tamoxifen®—maybe it's because you're still so young at heart," I kidded.

"I suggest adding in a mid-dose transdermal bioidentical estradiol to mitigate some of the symptoms, while staying on the Tamoxifen® (a controversial therapy mode, but one coming into usage occasionally). I'd taper you rapidly from 0.05 down to 0.0375, and then from 0.0375 or 0.05 to 0.025, and then imperceptively to zero over 2-3 years to coincide with the conclusion of your course of Tamoxifen®. I'd then switch you to raloxifen long term for both cancer prevention and your bones. With a Stage 1a1 tumor, I don't feel you'd be disadvantaging yourself. Check with your oncologist, though, and perhaps a GYN oncologist as well and think it over. Weigh the alternatives carefully. They are alternatives; since nothing else has helped with your symptoms, this has a good chance of success."

Shirley still wasn't convinced but "took it under advisement." Although her quality of life was excellent, the hot flashes and resultant insomnia (which had been unrelieved by vitamin E and even Effexor®) was taking its toll on her scholarly patience.

We talked at length about breast cancer, estrogens, and causality, and the data which showed no adverse effects for short-term estrogen therapy in breast cancer survivors.

Shirley returned 2 weeks later, not to discuss therapy, but with a yeast infection ("I used to get them before when I was married," she explained. "...Aahh, the wages of sin.")

She still wasn't sure about adding in the estradiol. I told her if she was still "hurting" and felt comfortable with the trial, to return "prn." In any case, we set a 2-month return appointment for follow up.

Shirley feels comfortable taking the vaginal estradiol supplementation and has elected for the time being not to add in transdermal systemic estrogens. She is much clearer, however, on the place for, and pros and cons of, estrogen supplementation in relation to breast cancer.

"I'm a pragmatist," she told me. "I'll give things another month. I take the Ambien® you give me for sleep every once in awhile and it's been helpful, but I don't want to get hooked on the stuff."

"I'm not really adverse to trying the estrogen—let's wait and see..."

*"It wasn't raining when Noah built the ark.".*
—Howard Ruff

# CHAPTER TEN

## BONE DENSITY ISSUES
(Also Called Osteoporosis)

According to the National Institutes of Health (NIH), of the 10 million Americans who suffer from osteoporosis, 8 million are woman over the age of 50. Additionally, an estimated <u>18 million</u> women with low bone mass have yet to be diagnosed or treated!

Osteoporosis is a devastating public health problem. Osteoporotic fractures are more common in women than heart attacks, stroke and breast cancer combined! The United States, blessed with an aging population, has the dubious distinction of being the world leader of fractures caused by this disease.

You don't want to get osteoporosis. It is a bad disease. The one year mortality after a hip fracture is 25-30% in women 65-80 and 40-50% over 80. Immobility bodes ill for older women.

You don't need to suffer from osteoporosis: this condition is <u>preventable</u>. Interventions with lifestyle modifications and medicinal measures preserve bone mass and prevent fractures.

Low bone mineral density (BMD) does not automatically confer fracture risk; only the need to follow up and put in place preventive measures (lifestyle and/or medicinal) to increase bone formation and minimize loss.

The idea here is to not let low bone density go and become a problem before you recognize it might be a problem-low bone density is a problem NOW. How to get it better?

### PATHOPHYSIOLOGY (HOW BONE WORKS)

Bone is dynamic, constantly changing. Bone "remodeling" is the process of bone formation and resorption (loss).

In the central core of bones, cells called osteoblasts promote bone formation by creating a collagen (connective tissue) mesh which becomes calcified, resulting in mineralized bone. Cellular osteoclasts promote bone resorption by the production of enzymes that dissolve old bone mineral and proteins.

"Away with the old and in with the new" (So long as not too much "old" is thrown away, and there's enough "new" to replace it!)

Normally, bone resorption is balanced by new bone formation. Bone loss occurs when there is an imbalance between bone removal and replacement, leading to a decrease in bone strength and increase in risk for fracture.

Bone mass increases throughout childhood and during one's 20s. As women approach midlife and menopause, bone loss begins to accelerate. Additionally, the period of greatest bone loss in women is that time around and immediately after menopause. When women discontinue hormone therapy, bone loss is accelerated, similar to that seen just after menopause. The exact rate of this acceleration depends on lifestyle and risk factors (discussed below). The decline in estrogen levels appears to be the predominant factor influencing increased bone loss in women.

## RISK FACTORS FOR OSTEOPOROSIS

What are risk factors for excessive bone loss?

The greatest influence on a person's maximal bone mass (and loss) is heredity. Black and brown women have higher BMD than White and Asian women, a difference that suggests genetic influence.

Several lifestyle factors may affect your risk of developing osteoporosis:

1. Nutrition:

After peak bone mass is attained in adulthood, "proper nutrition" (c'mon: protein, fruit, veggies, grains, some but not too much meat...) is essential.

Additionally, calcium and vitamin D have important roles in bone metabolism. Poor nutrition and chronic lack of calcium and vitamin D (found in vitamin supplements and sunlight) are important risk factors.

2. Physical Activity:

Regular exercise is associated with reduced fracture risk. Conversely, a sedentary lifestyle and periods of prolonged bed rest increase risk. Exercise stimulates osteoblast (bone replacement) activity.

3. Cigarette Smoking:

Compared with a non-smoker, smokers lose bone more rapidly, have lower bone mass and reach menopause an average of 2 years earlier.

4. Alcohol consumption:

Heavy alcohol consumption (over 7 "drinks" per week, or generally in excess of one drink per day) has detrimental effects on BMD. Additionally, excessive alcohol increases the risk of falls and hip fracture. Moderate alcohol consumption, however (an average of 1 drink a day or less) may lower the risk for hip fractures.

There is definitely a hormonal influence on bone mass in women. The drop in estrogen production accompanying menopause is a likely explanation for the increased bone resorption (loss) seen in women compared to men after age 50.

Various medical conditions and medications are associated with bone loss. These "secondary causes" of osteoporosis in young women include chronically low estrogen levels, hyperthyroidism or taking too high a dose of thyroid replacement, anticonvulsant medications, and especially the use of oral glucocorticoids ("steroids") for therapy of asthma, rheumatoid arthritis and some chronic obstructive lung conditions. Additionally, the prolonged (greater than 5-6 months) use of medications to suppress endometriosis or shrink fibroids (e.g., Lupron®) or the use of depo-medroxyprogesterone acetate ("DepoProvera®") for contraception or other reasons for over 6-12 months is also associated with premature loss of bone density.

EVALUATION: How to tell if you're OK or not.
Physical Signs of Osteoporosis:
    Loss of height in older women is a sign of vertebral fracture. Acute or chronic back pain or easily breaking bones from a not-too-severe fall in the post menopause should raise your physician's suspicion.
BMD Measurement:
    There are several methods of measuring bone density; a simple "x-ray" is not one of them.
    These may be broken down into two categories: central and peripheral.
    A "central" (lumbar spine, hip) bone density is the only way to accurately follow your bone mineral density.
    The technical "gold standard" of central measurement is "Dual Energy X-Ray Absorptionetry" ("DXA," more commonly referred to as "DEXA"). The total hip and lumbar spine is the preferred site for BMD testing especially in women older than 60. Computerized tomography ("CT") can also be used accurately, especially for bone density determinations of the lower spine.
    Values are reported either as a "Z-score" or a "T-score." A T-score measures how your bones compare to a "...normal young adult"; a Z-score measures how you compare to an average woman of the same age and ethnicity. Scores are measured in "standard deviations" above and below "the mean," or average. The most meaningful comparison is the T-score. A T-score of -1.0 or better is "normal"; a score of -1.0 to -1.5 indicates mild bone loss (osteopenia); -1.5 to -2, moderate osteopenia; -2 to -2.5, severe osteopenia; and less than -2.5, osteoporosis.

How often to repeat bone density measurements?

If you are already osteoporotic and on therapy, a repeat in 1 year is probably appropriate to make sure your loss is stabilized and to assess whether a combined medical therapy (using more than one preparation) may be warranted.

Usually bone densities should be rechecked approximately every 2 years during initial follow-up of women with moderate or severe osteopenia and later follow-up of women with osteoporosis. In untreated women with mild or even moderate osteopenia, DEXA testing is generally not useful until at least 3 years have passed.

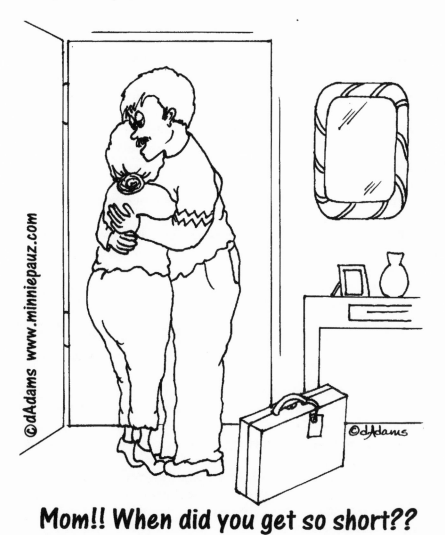

Mom!! When did you get so short??

So called "peripheral bone density measurement" of the wrist or calcaneus (heel) are good for screening those women who may have lowered bone density and therefore may be candidates for a DEXA. The results of a peripheral bone density are not as precise and cannot be used to diagnose osteoporosis or follow response to therapy. If your peripheral bone density looks OK (-1.0 to -1.5 or higher) you should be fine; if it's lower than -1.5, a DEXA should be done.

Biochemical Markers:

Blood and urine tests have some, but limited usage in the diagnosis and treatment of osteopenia and osteoporosis.

A few urine assays (Pyrilinks D, "NTX," and "CTX") are available which more or less measure the amount of calcium loss via urinary excretion, giving an idea of how much bone is being lost and a better understanding of whether your medication is working to prevent excessive loss. The test may be helpful if you are severely osteopenic or osteoporotic to help measure the effectiveness of your medications to limit excessive breakdown.

## WHO SHOULD BE TESTED AND HOW?

Following in outline form is a listing of who should be tested, what type of test, and when:

DEXA

1. All women over age 65, especially those not on estrogen, a SERM or other bone-protective medication.
2. Peri- or newly post-menopausal women (± age 45-60) with one or more of the following risk factors:
   a. One or more first generation relatives with osteoporosis
   b. Very slender and Caucasian or Asian
   c. Slender and a smoker and/or excessive alcohol history
   d  History of prolonged drug therapy with corticosteroids, anticonvulsants or DepoProvera® 1 year or greater, or Lupron® for 6 months or more.
   e. One or more fractures caused by anything other than a forceful accident
3. Younger women (approximately age 30-45) with history of long-term therapy with corticosteroids, anti-endometriosis or fibroid-shrinking medication (e.g., Lupron®) or prolonged exposure to DepoProvera®.
4. Younger women (approximately age 35-45) with history of prolonged amenorrhea (no periods) related to bulimia, anorexia, competitive athletics, or a very low Body Mass Index ("BMI" under 12).

Peripheral (e.g. heel) bone density has great usage as a screening procedure and can be used for:

1. Peri/newly menopausal women electing not to take hormonal supplementation.
2. All women discontinuing HRT, within a year of stopping.
3. Younger women with some of the risk factors noted above who are not able to get a central bone density measurement.
4. Anyone concerned about their bone density.

A peripheral bone density test, by ultrasound or x-ray, is a screening procedure only. A central (DEXA) measurement is necessary to accurately diagnose osteoporosis and determine follow-up therapy. A screening density is useful to confirm normalcy. If it shows possible osteopenia (T-score less than -1.0; certainly less than -1.5) a central measurement should be performed.

## FOLLOW-UP:

How often, if you're normal? How often, if you're not?
1. Peri/post-menopausal peripheral screens with no risk factors: screen every 5 years is fine.
2. Peri/post-menopausal DEXA for risk factors (see above) with T-values -1.5 or better: DEXA every 5 years or peripheral screen every 3 years.
3. Peri/post-menopausal DEXA with osteopenia (-1.5 to -2.5): DEXA every 2 years.
4. Patients with osteoporosis (T-score less than -2.5): yearly until stable; then every 2-3 years if no longer osteoporotic.
5. Women over 65: Initial DEXA. If better than -1.5, repeat every 5 years; if -1.5 to -2.5, every 2-3 years; if osteoporotic, repeat every 1-2 years.

Remember, of course: If you are significantly osteopenic (worse than -2) or osteoporotic, you must be exercising, taking calcium and vitamin D (and possibly magnesium) and using something (1 or 2 things) to help prevent additional loss.

## HOW TO BUILD NEW BONE AND PREVENT LOSS OF WHAT YOU HAVE

Remember that bone is dynamic. You've gotta keep building it up and prevent excessive breakdown.

It's really not that hard! Here are some basic "build-up" tips.
1. A "balanced diet" is important for bone development as well as general health. Eat more fruit and veggies and minimize consumption of fats (You've heard this before from me-probably won't be the last time!) You need enough protein too! (especially as you age-over 70 or 75). Protein supplements are OK if your diet doesn't provide.
2. You need calcium and vitamin D (and perhaps magnesium). Below age 65: 1200 mg calcium (take in two or three divided doses). At least 800

I.U. of vitamin D per day and approximately 600 mg of magnesium. If you're over 65, increase the calcium to 1500 mg (the vitamin D and magnesium can stay the same or go up a bit also). Sources for calcium: any calcium supplement is fine (read the label). One glass of milk is approximately 300 mg; 8 oz of yogurt approximately 415 mg; 2 cup ice cream equals 90 mg; 1 serving cheese approximately 200 mg. Interestingly, one serving of broccoli, collards, bok choy, kale, turnip greens, sardines and tofu with calcium sulfate all supply 200-300 mg of calcium.

3.  Exercise (!) raises its head too, especially weight-bearing (lifting, carrying of light/moderate weights). 15-45 minutes 4-6 times per week. The exercise "mobilizes" the calcium and gets it into the bones.

4.  Fluoride can be helpful too. If your community doesn't have fluoridated water, consider a supplement if fluoride is not in your multi-vitamin (1 mg every other day is sufficient).

You can do all the things to build-up bone density, but if you're "genetically challenged" in the bone department, you've also got to prevent excessive bone breakdown..

If you have a family history of osteoporosis or other risk factors and a BMD shows you to be low (T-score less than 1.5) it's probably important to do something to prevent excessive bone catabolism (or breakdown). Usually one of the following is sufficient, but if there is further loss, or if you are already osteoporotic (T-score less than 2.5), I'd recommend combining two of these.

## SUBSTANCES KNOWN TO PREVENT EXCESSIVE BONE LOSS:

1.  Estrogens. Makes no difference whether oral or transdermal, whether synthetic or bioidentical. 0.3 mg of conjugated estrogens, 0.5 mg of estradiol and a 0.025 mg estradiol patch are all minimal doses known to protect against excessive bone breakdown.

2.  SERMs: Raloxifene (Evista®) is the only presently available SERM, and numerous studies have shown its beneficial effect on preventing bone loss. New SERMs coming out soon should do fine also.

3.  Bisphosphonates: Presently available are alendronate (Fosamax®), risedronate (Actonel®), and etidionate (Didronel®). The first two are somewhat easier to use and are available in both daily and once-weekly dosages. These are mildly complicated to take (must be taken in the morning, ½ hour before any food in your stomach, with a full glass of water, and you can't lie down for ½ hour). They can also cause stomach upset in women with sensitive GI tracts. But most women tolerate it just fine.

4. Calcitonin® nasal spray: Also has a good track record for preventing bone loss, but not used as much nowadays since the bisphosphonates (which are more effective) have come out.
5. Testosterone: Also quite effective in preventing bone loss. (That's why the rate of osteoporosis in men is only 20% of what it is in women.) After a pass or two through the liver, testosterone is broken down into estradiol, which occupies receptor sites in the bone. If you're not on estrogens, however, you have to monitor testosterone levels carefully so as not to get signs of excessive male characteristics (like hair growth, oily skin, etc.).

**SUBSTANCES PURPORTED TO PREVENT BONE LOSS** (but with... "softer science"). These probably help, but not as surely as those listed above.
1. DHEA (dose 25 mg twice daily). DHEA is broken down into testosterone, among other things.
2. Statins (Zocor®, Mevacor®, etc.). Studies are conflicting here: some show bone protection, others not necessarily. Statins certainly do not hurt, and probably help prevent excessive bone loss.
3. Progesterone (oral micronized progesterone, or Prometrium®; not synthetic progestins). Like estrogen deficiency, the progesterone deficiency experienced during menopause has been found to possibly contribute to bone loss. Some studies (not all) have shown that oral micronized progesterone (Prometrium®) has a bone-enhancing effect, but one which is less potent than estrogen. Progesterone skin cream has not been shown to help with BMD, but it does help diminish hot flashes in many women.

**COMBINATION THERAPIES**
Combining HRT/ERT or a SERM with a bisphosphonate (Actonel®, Fosamax®, or Didronel®) is probably the best combination for preventing bone loss in significantly affected individuals. And adding some testosterone or DHEA certainly wouldn't hurt!

**Treatment for Osteoporosis:**
Until recently there was no good, fairly rapid, aggressive therapy to build new bone for men and women with significant osteoporosis. This changed in 2002 with the approval of teriparatide (Forteo®), a synthetic human parathyroid hormone extract made by Eli Lily & Co. Forteo® has been shown to reduce new vertebral fractures by 65% and hip and wrist fractures by more than 50%, as it restructures the micro architecture of the bone itself.

Although it appears to be the next best thing to homogenized milk, Forteo® increases bone resorption (loss) as well as bone formation, so it is best combined with another "anti-resorptive" agent.

The down side of parathyroid hormone is that it is given as a daily injection and is hugely expensive. It is, however, the only agent which will build significant amounts of new bone, giving new hope to those women with severe osteoporosis.

These medications are not something to "try by yourself at home." An M.D. or qualified health professional (preferably a gynecologist or knowledgeable internist or family physician) should help you fashion your best therapeutic approach.

Drug therapies and lifestyle adjustments are hugely under-utilized in post-menopausal women, most of whom have never had a bone density determination of any sort.

Most women are not actively pursuing lifestyle or medicinal approaches to maintain their bone density. A recent study in New England showed that only 20% of elderly people who had a hip fracture were subsequently treated for osteoporosis!

Hey! Like so much else in this book, this isn't rocket science. Eat healthy! Exercise! Take enough calcium and vitamin D. Have at least a screening BMD around menopause time (or before, if you're in a high risk group).

The best therapy for osteoporosis?? PREVENTION!!

## RICHA'S STORY

Richa Adzhbanian first came to see me about hormone replacement therapy. She'd gone through menopause early, at age 41-42 and was started on hormonal supplementation (PremPro®) by her gynecologist. This helped considerably with her insomnia and hot flashes, but she was still low energy, with very little libido. Because of this, and worried about breast cancer (her 77-year-old mother had recently been diagnosed), Richa had stopped her HRT six months before, at age 46 and now was miserable, with insomnia, day and night hot flashes, poor memory, low energy and basically a zero sexual desire.

In getting her history, I discovered that, in addition to a long history of a teen and twenties eating disorder ("I got down to a body mass index of 9 and didn't have a period for over a year.") Richa had been a cigarette smoker and fairly heavy drinker in her 20s and early 30s. In addition, I discovered that her mom, although never having had a bone density study, had lost over 2" of height in the past several years. Richa herself was slender at 5'5" tall and 122 lbs.

Having already taken hormones for 4 years, Richa was quite concerned about an increased risk of breast cancer. She was somewhat relieved when I informed her that with only one first generation relative with breast cancer, especially at age 77, her risk was not substantially elevated. Additionally, the fact that she experienced a relatively early menopause conferred a degree of protection.

After some discussion of alternatives, we decided on a 0.0375 estradiol patch (I usually prescribe the Vivelle-Dot®, which because it is approximately ¼ the size of other patches, is very patient friendly). I added 200 mg of micronized progesterone (Prometrium®) to be taken at night, to further help with sleep and hot flashes, plus some bioidentical transdermal testosterone lotion (5 mg per day initially, then going to 5 mg every other day) to help with her libido and low energy.

And I arranged for a DEXA later that week.

Richa returned 3 weeks later. Her pre-therapy salivary testosterone had come back low (not surprisingly) at 15.9, but she was now sleeping and feeling somewhat better on her HRT.

The biggest news, however, was her DEXA result, which showed her to be severely osteopenic/early osteoporotic with a T-score of -2.3 average for the lower spine, and -2.6 for the femoral neck (the weakest part of the hip).

"This is definitely down for a woman only in her 40s, but not really unexpected, given your history," I explained.

We reviewed her options. Upon investigation, it turned out that she had been taking no calcium but was exercising 3-4 times per week. She was rarely in the sun and her multivitamin had only 400 I.U. of vitamin D. I suggested a calcium supplement containing 600 mg of calcium, 300 mg of magnesium and 400 I.U. of vitamin D and asked her to take 2 per day, as well as adding 15 minutes of floor weights and machines to her workouts.

"I feel confident that the HRT, especially with the added testosterone will help slow down your bone loss," I counseled.

The next question was whether or not to add in a second agent. With Richa's quite significant bone loss at a relatively young age, we decided to "take out all the stops" and add in Actonel® 35 mg per week, so long as she was able to tolerate it.

When her hot flashes did not initially come under control, I increased her estradiol to 0.05 mg for several months, slowly tapering back to 0.0375 six months later. Over the next year, Richa slowly trimmed off an additional 5-10% of her patch every month or two so that in a year she was down to 0.025 mg and free of symptoms.

"I like the balance of my present regimen," Richa told me at a follow-up check. "I'd really like to stop my estrogens, but stay on testosterone. Is that possible? I don't want to grow a mustache!"

We decided on a 4-6 month taper-down on the patch, slowly adding in Evista®, first at 30 mg and then the full dose of 60 mg halfway through her final taper. We followed salivary testosterone closely, keeping it in a 30-50 mg range (Richa decreased her lotion to 0.4 cc every other day).

A couple of Pyrilinks assays (urine test that measures bone resorption) confirmed minimal urinary calcium loss. Richa found it very hard to wait a full 2 years to recheck her bone density. A repeat DEXA 20 months after her first showed her hip T-score to have improved to -2.4 and the spine to -2.1. We were headed in the right direction.

Now (4 years later), repeat DEXA shows a T-score of -2.1 for the femoral neck and a stable -1.9 for her lumbar spine. Richa has elected to discontinue the Actonel® ("I'm taking too many meds!"), and we'll follow this change with a couple of urinary calcium assays and another bone density in 2 years. She dropped back on the testosterone to 0.2 cc every other evening (because of a bit of a mustache) and had added in DHEA 25 mg twice daily.

She is doing well!

*If I had known I was going to live this long, I would have taken better care of myself.*

—Jazz pianist Eubie Blake, upon
reaching the age of 100

# CHAPTER ELEVEN

## PRESERVING YOUR HEALTH
The Heart; Diabetes; Cancer;
The Exercise Connection.
"Living Well Into Later Life"

It all revolves around this, doesn't it?

Many of us are lucky enough to have been born with good genes not subjecting us to increased risk of hypertension, heart disease, diabetes, etc. Some of us were raised by parents who were health conscious and kept us away from fats and fast foods and somehow prepared us for the joys of fresh fruits and vegetables and exemplified the ideas of fitness and regular exercise.

But most of us weren't.

So, what can you do <u>now</u>? (No sense crying over past spilled milkshakes.)

Let me again be clear. What follows really works and is honest-to-God true, but a lot of it would probably fall under the heading of "tough love" or "you don't get something for nothing."

Metabolife® and other forms of ephedra, "speed," any "diet pill," or fad diet you'd care to mention is what I mean by "something for nothing." Easy to do and almost guaranteed to lose you 20-30 lbs. or more. And equally guaranteed that you will gain all of it back (plus 5-10 lbs., usually) within the next 2 years and certainly be no healthier or happier in the bargain.

The following is written to guide you into "living well into later life." Let's start out with a guide to your "annual exam" and then go through the major health issues of diminished memory/Alzheimer's, diabetes, cardiovascular disease, cancer prevention and detection, and weight gain. Another important issue, osteoporosis, was the topic of the last chapter.

The common thread to most of this, as you shall see, involves our old friends, diet and exercise.

What should you expect as part of your "annual physical exam"? Well, an exam, of course (covering blood pressure, pulse, head, chest, heart, breasts, belly, and pelvic exam). But what other evaluations should be part of an "annual"?

Here is your "annual exam checklist" of tests and their timing. Feel free to copy it or tear it out and bring it to your primary care practitioner (and demand it of your HMO).

1.  Pap Smear: Every year up to age 50, although every 2 years is probably OK for women in their 40s who have had several consecutive negative smears in the previous 5-10 years; every 2 years in your 50s and every 3 years after age 60 in women who are not being followed for a cervical abnormality.

2.  Mammograms: Every 2 years after 40; yearly after 50. If strong family history of breast cancer, probably start at age 30-35 and go yearly after 40.

3.  Occult blood in the stool (also called "hemoccult"; "occult blood" in medical parlance means originating from somewhere other than the place of exit): Yearly after age 50. If strong family history of colon cancer, start at age 40. The necessity for this test may be modified if you are having sigmoidoscopy or colonoscopy.

4.  "Blood Count" (CBC or hemogram): Every 3-5 years.

5.  "Metabolic Panel" (including fasting blood sugar, liver and kidney tests, etc.): Every 5 years.

6.  TSH (sensitive thyroid evaluation): Should be done on all peri-menopausal women and every 5 years thereafter.

7.  Lipids (in women without abnormal cholesterol): Every 5 years.

8.  Homocysteine: Every 3 years in women with increased stress or increased fats in their diet; every 5 years as a screen along with lipids.

9.  C-Reactive Protein (CRP): Do whenever lipid profile is poor; otherwise include in 5 year screen along with lipids.

10. Colonoscopy: Every 10 years after age 50 unless strong family history of colon cancer; then every 5 years starting at age 40-45. Sigmoidoscopy is a "poor relative" of colonoscopy as it evaluates only the lower third of the colon (but is easier to perform and is better than nothing. Also, most cancers do start in the lower part of the colon).

11. DEXA: The complete hip and spine bone density test. After age 65 in all women, especially if not taking an anti-resorptive agent or otherwise "at risk"; earlier as per guidelines outlined in Chapter 10.

12. BMI: A "body mass index" or BMI should be done periodically, especially if you're overweight. A BMI of 25 or lower is what you want. Risk of diabetes and heart disease rises after that, especially if your BMI is over 30 or 35.

13. EKG. Electrocardiogram, an electrical recording of heart function. Good to get one at or shortly after menopause. Repeat later only if needed.

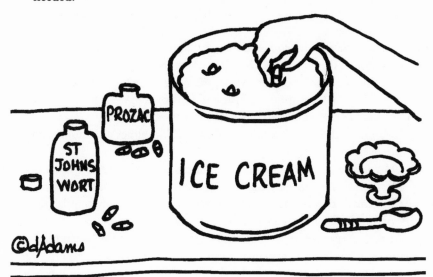

# How to eat ice cream without the guilt!

### Memory Enhancement/Alzheimer's Prevention

Ginkgo biloba is marketed for use as a treatment to improve memory, attention and cognitive function. Some studies have shown a modest improvement in memory at a dose of 50 mg (25 mg twice daily) and some studies suggest an increase of blood flow to the brain.

Unfortunately, other controlled studies show no improved results over placebo. Unfortunately also, when an independent federal laboratory recently tested 10 brands of ginkgo off the shelf, only 3 were found to contain approximately the amount advertised on the label. One had no ginkgo at all! One had an excessively large dose and the other four were significantly below the dose.

*Caveat emptor!* It may help. Probably doesn't hurt (don't take if you are on blood thinners or if you regularly take high doses of ibuprofen or aspirin).

(Again, remember: frequent, vigorous exercise probably improves blood flow to your brain much more than 50 mg of ginkgo a day.)

A recent large study suggests that the long term use of small amounts of aspirin and/or the use of other NSAIDs (e.g., ibuprofen, naprosyn, etc.) may reduce the risk of Alzheimer's by 30-40%.

Several scientists have noted that anti-oxidants (especially when combined with a low fat diet!) lower the risk of Alzheimer's disease. Although anti-oxidants (vitamins B, C, E, beta carotene, flavinoids) can certainly be taken in pill form, it is the dietary intake of these substances that does the best work.

Overweight elderly women are more likely than those who stay trim to be stricken by Alzheimer's. Data are now strong enough to recommend a dietary strategy for reducing the Alzheimer's disease risk that includes low fat intake and high consumption of fish and anti-oxidants, along with vitamin E, folic acid, and vitamin B6 and B12 supplements.

Two major dietary patterns that relate to Alzheimer's disease have been identified:

One, labeled "low anti-oxidant, high-fat" consists of large amounts of red meat, processed meat, French fries, refined grains (food from milled flour and corn), sweets, eggs, nuts, margarine, cold breakfast cereals, high fat dairy products, fried chicken and high energy drinks.

At the other extreme, a "high anti-oxidant, low-fat" diet includes fruits, vegetables, whole grains, tomatoes, seafood and poultry.

In a recent study, the risk of developing Alzheimer's disease among those who followed the high anti-oxidant, low fat diet during mid/adult life and beyond (after age 40) was only ⅓ that of people who consumed the less healthy diet!

A possible explanation for this has been offered by Dr. Robert Friedland of Case Western Reserve University. He postulates that, "For over 99% of human history, we consumed a diet lower in fat and higher in vitamins and anti-oxidants than is consumed today in developed countries. The genes we have now were selected for because of their adaptive value in this earlier period of hunting and gathering.

"It may be that Alzheimer's disease is, in part, a disease of modern life, similar to arteriosclerosis, hypertension and diabetes, reflecting an imbalance between our current lifestyle and that in which our genes were selected."

Bottom line for Alzheimer's disease prevention: high anti-oxidant, low fat diet with vitamins C, E, and mega-B supplementation; regular exercise; regular (daily or every other day) use of 80-160 mg aspirin or 200 mg ibuprofen. Estrogens also may help, but Alzheimer's prevention shouldn't be the only reason for taking long-term estrogen supplementation.

## DIABETES.

Even people without a genetic predisposition can get diabetes, but, as often as not, it "runs in the family."

A big question here is: does it run in the family because of true genetic reasons or because your parents, sisters, aunts, grandparents, etc. all have the same poor dietary habits and lack exercise?

That's the key to diabetes prevention: diet and exercise. The findings of study after study implicate excessive body fat as the risk factor most predictive of Type II or "adult-onset" diabetes. A great majority of cases might be prevented by losing weight, exercising regularly and vigorously, eating a "proper diet," abstaining from smoking and taking limited amounts of alcohol (yes-an average of ½ to 1 drink per day helps prevent diabetes). Of these measures, weight control seems to offer the most benefit.

If you have two or more of the following risk factors, ask your doctor to test you for diabetes: High blood pressure, high cholesterol (especially high LDLs with lower HDLs), smoking, overweight (body mass index over 25), family history of diabetes, history of having very large babies-especially if you are of Hispanic, African-American, Native American or Pacific Island descent.

**AN AFFAIR OF THE HEART** (...Well, the cardiovascular system, to be specific; all the blood vessels in your heart, lungs, kidneys, brain, and elsewhere)

Heart disease and hypertension are far and away the biggest killers of women-way more than all cancers combined. "The biggies."

Wanna be healthy in this area? Yeah, of course it helps to be born with the right genetics and to have had parents who pounded good nutrition down your sweet-tooth-lined little childhood gullet.

But now you're 40. What are the risks? How do you practice prevention and stay healthy? And what are the most valuable tools to see how you're doing?

Risk factors

It's a good idea for all women in midlife to be tested periodically for "markers" of elevated cardiovascular disease (CVD) risk and these tests will be more specifically discussed a bit later.

Obviously, a strong family history of heart disease and/or hypertension is a risk factor for you and an added reason to "lead the healthy life." The family history connection may be a primary one because of genetically-inherited vascular problems, or may be secondary to abnormal lipid metabolism. Obesity, lack of exercise, high fat/processed/fast food diet and smoking are obvious "risk factors."

Abnormal lipids, especially elevated low density lipoprotein (LDL) cholesterol and triglycerides and lowered high density lipoproteins (HDL) also may be genetic or nutritional.

Vascular spasms contribute to risk. Cigarette smoking and stress both promote spasm and therefore are risk factors.

At highest risk are people who have what is called the "metabolic syndrome." Metabolic syndrome is diagnosed when a woman has three or more of the following: abdominal obesity (waist of over 40"); elevated triglycerides of 150 or more; high density lipoprotein (HDL) level of below 50; blood pressure over 130/85 or fasting glucose of 110 or above. Individuals with metabolic syndrome are much more likely than others to develop diabetes and cardiovascular disease and have increased mortality from all causes and CVD in particular.

In perhaps one-half of cases of early vascular disease, a positive family history of this is the apparent cause even when there are no other risk factors (such as physical inactivity, smoking, abnormal lipids, hypertension, obesity, diabetes).

New information strongly implicates abnormal homocysteine metabolism, the result of a genetic deficiency in "cystathione beta-synthetase," an enzyme which converts homocysteine to the more benign cysteine. Deficiency of this enzyme results in increased concentrations in body fluids of homocysteine and its dietary precursor, the amino acid methionine. High levels of homocysteine have been found to be an independent risk factor for arteriosclerosis, especially in persons under the age of 55.

### Diagnosis:

The traditional laboratory markers of CVD risk in midlife women include elevated levels of LDLs, low levels of HDLs and high triglycerides, especially if combined with an elevated fasting blood sugar. These parameters should be routinely checked during peri-menopause and at least every 5 years.

In recent years, several new markers have been found that may prove critical in the assessment of CVD risk:

1. C-Reactive Protein (or CRP) is a marker for systemic inflammation. Researchers have long speculated that arteriosclerosis is an inflammatory process. An elevated CRP of over 4 (probably over 2), especially if confirmed on repeat testing, is a strong predictor for risk of developing CVD. In a recent large study, women with the highest levels of CRP had a fivefold increase in the risk of developing CVD and a sevenfold increase in the risk of having a heart attack or stroke, compared with those who had the lowest levels of CRP. Increased levels of CRP predicted these events even among apparently low risk women.

2. Homocysteine: Elevated levels of this amino acid have been correlated with arterial damage, blood clotting, myocardial infarction, stroke, etc. Blood homocysteine levels increase at menopause.

3. Fibrinogen: The body depends on this protein for proper blood clotting. However, high levels of fibrinogen can lead to hardened arteries and accumulation of plaque. Fibrinogen is a highly predictive marker for reduced elasticity of arteries.

If you are at high risk because of the risk factors already discussed or abnormal lab results, ask your health care practitioner about an "exercise stress test" electrocardiogram, which is sensitive in picking up CVD. If, however, you are athletically "in shape," the stress test may not pick up a blockage. In that case, inquire about a "thallium stress test" which can detect CVD that may otherwise be missed.

So, if you are at higher risk, what do you do about it?

## Diet and Cardio Protection

Despite its central role in the prevention of coronary artery disease, diet is frequently obscured by the often-impressive effects of medications.

You are what you eat! Face up, folks, you can't eat at McDonald's™ or Taco Bell™ and snack on donuts and expect to be a healthy, happy camper into middle and older age.

The American Heart Association and the National Cholesterol Education Program, Adult Treatment Panel, have recently reviewed their guidelines and have reached several clear conclusions:

Emphasis is on an overall balanced diet that includes a variety of foods: 5-6 servings per day of whole grains and complex carbohydrates (e.g., whole grain breads, pasta, healthy cereal, potatoes, legumes: peas and beans) along with 5 or more servings of fruits and veggies. (A high nutrient-to-calorie ratio and rich in fiber!)

The new guidelines place a new emphasis on fish-particularly fatty fish such as tuna and salmon, and on other products that provide a balanced set of nutrients such as legumes (peas and beans), lean meat and non-fat or low fat dairy products.

Major emphasis is also on maintaining a healthy body weight-specifically by matching caloric intake to physical activity level.

Recommendations for maintaining a desirable lipoprotein profile include limiting saturated fats and transfatty acids (often shown on food labels as "hydrogenated" fats) which raise LDL cholesterol, such as are found in baked goods, fried foods, margarine and "fast foods."

Two or more servings of fish per week (especially salmon) is recommended as well as nuts, flax seed, soy bean and canola oils.

Emphasis on maintaining a normal blood pressure is actualized by limiting salt and alcohol, avoiding weight gain, and (again) eating fruits and veggies and lowfat dairy products.

As far as supplements go, B vitamins, folic acid and "long-chain omega-3 fatty acids" (found in fish oils) have been shown to reduce coronary events.

### The Exercise Connection

I'm not going to get carried away here. By now I'm sure you already know the necessity for and the benefits of exercise!

Almost daily (at least 4-5 times per week). 20-60 minutes of exercise (including weights) that causes you to sweat, be at least a bit out of breath, and causes your pulse to rise at least 40-60 beats above baseline is the goal. (Of course, check with your personal physician prior to any significant exercise program.)

The reward? A previously sedentary individual can reasonably expect a modest, yet helpful 5% rise in HDLs by adopting an aerobic exercise program, not to mention the body sculpting and increased mental acuity that exercise provides.

Additionally, at the very least, a regular exercise program can help you develop good collateral circulation, so that if you do block off a major artery to your heart, you'll at least have a few alternative routes or detours for blood to take so you won't die right off, can have your bypass, and then better clean up your act so you can "live to see another day."

### Medications and Treatment for Abnormal Lipids, Elevated CRP and Homocysteine

1. Lipid Modifiers: If you've got abnormal lipids secondary to genetic or dietary factors (or both), more than a band-aid are a group of drugs known as "lipid modifiers." There are several classes of these medications, all of them useful. The newest, most well known and most effective are a group of medications known as "statins." There are several medications in this category, one essentially as useful as another. Your physician's selection has to do with which one s(he) has most experience with, or which one your insurance plan covers. Lovastatin, atorvastatin (Lipitor®), fluvastatin (Leascol®), pravastatin (Pravachol®), and simvastatin (Zocor®) are in this group.

   Other lipid modifiers are niacin (best as Niaspan®, an extended release version, or niacin combined with lovastatin, known as Advicon®); medications that modify bile acids (cholestryamine, Welchol®, Colestid®), and "fibrates" (Gemfibrozil® and fenofibrate or Tricor®).

Niacin is an unsung hero of cardiovascular risk reductic ‿ can be used along with statins. Flushing (similar to hot flashes), however, is a major hassle with all but the extended release version (Niaspan®). Time-release niacin is also available in over-the-counter form.

The bile acid modifiers can also be used with statins. Fibrates are impressive in lowering triglycerides and boosting HDL cholesterol and especially good in diabetic patients.

Lipid lowering experts frequently use combination drug therapy, especially in patients with low HDLs and high triglycerides or patients who respond only modestly to statins.

Statins, due to their proven risk reduction in women are the treatment of choice for high cholesterol and have been shown to dramatically reduce levels of cholesterol along with a significantly beneficial effect in reducing coronary heart disease events. The effects of statins and HRT, or SERMs, are additive in lowering LDL cholesterol and raising HDL cholesterol.

With the exception of over-the-counter niacin, whichever one or combinations of medications that you use is going to cost somebody $100-$250 a month. That, of course, brings you back to the protective importance of lifestyle changes (diet and exercise) and 80 mg aspirin/day.

2.  SERMs

SERMs are emerging as another class of medications with potential beneficial effects on lipids. Studies with raloxifene (Evista®), a presently available SERM, and others, have shown that they are capable of reducing LDL levels and fibrinogen (fibrinogen is a protein in the body that clots blood; too much fibrinogen means a greater risk of problem-causing blood clots).

3.  Therapy of Elevated Homocysteine (homocysteine level 14 or greater)

Elevated homocysteine levels are thought to increase inflammation of the arteries, leading to more arterial blood clots.

Treatment with a combination of folic acid (1 mg per day), vitamin B12 (400 mcg or more per day) and vitamin B6 or pyridoxine (10 mg or more per day) significantly ameliorates the adverse effects on blood vessels from increased homocysteine levels. Not all doctors are aware of the homocysteine connection (or its treatment), however.

4.  Therapy of elevated C-Reactive Protein (CRP, level of 4 or greater)

Elevated CRP level is an indicator of risk that plaque buildup in arteries may rupture and cause blood clots. Patients with an elevated CRP should have a homocysteine level test and, if elevated, be treated appropriately.

An elevated CRP in the absence of abnormal lipids should increase awareness to actualize dietary changes and keep a closer laboratory track of cardiovascular health, perhaps with additional testing (stress EKG, echocardiogram, etc.)

5. Cardiac Friendly Dietary Supplements for Midlife Women

What do I advise? Vitamin C 500-1000 mg per day, vitamin E 400 mg per day, a "mega B" supplement, folic acid 400 mcg a day or more, and calcium/magnesium/vitamin D as described in Chapter 10. Glucosamine and chondroitin may be helpful for the joints; ginkgo may be helpful for memory. Flax seed oil/omega-3 fatty acid supplement.

Again, dietary sources are best: fish, fish oils, chicken, whole grains, fresh fruits and veggies (especially deep greens), legumes, potatoes, pasta, rice.

## THYROID

Thyroid dysfunction can happen at any time, but is especially common in midlife. All peri-menopausal women should be tested for abnormal thyroid function. Thyroid levels are best checked with a sensitive TSH (thyroid stimulating hormone) level, but other tests may be necessary.

An FTI or "free thyroxin index" should also be performed if you are taking hormone replacement therapy.

Additionally, if fatigue is your issue and TSH is normal, it may be appropriate to check for thyromicroglobulins and anti-thyroid antibodies as part of your workup (see Chapter 16 for more detail).

Disruption in the normal menstrual cycle is common when thyroid dysfunction is present. Both too high (hyperthyroid) and too low (hypothyroid) lead to menstrual abnormalities. Alterations in thyroid hormone levels exert significant effects on a woman's hormone production and metabolism and even on sex hormone binding globulin (SHBG) levels. (Hyperthyroidism increases SHBG levels.)

Hyperthyroidism is most commonly associated with infrequent or absent menses, while hypothyroidism is most often associated with heavy and/or long periods, but sometimes may cause lack of menses as well.

Weight gain, fatigue, abnormal menses, hyperlipidemia (abnormally high lipids) and constipation are all signs of hypothyroidism.

Thyroid replacement is either with levothyroxine (Synthroid®; Levoxyl®) or Armor Thyroid® (made from porcine-pig-thyroid tissue). Levothyroxine is usually used, but if you are not responding properly, speak with your health care practitioner about the use of porcine thyroid.

A small pearl: don't take thyroid at the same time as soy products-they inhibit absorption.

## WEIGHT GAIN:

Weight gain is a normal accompaniment of the midlife passage. The reasons are multiple:

1. As we age, our "motor" slows down. We simply metabolize less calories.
2. Our lifestyle tends to get more sedentary as we age.
3. We tend to substitute food for other things we used to do more of (like sex, strenuous activities, etc.)
4. We eat out more often.
5. Some of the medications we now take tend to add a pound or three.

Weight is simply a matter of addition and subtraction. Calories in and calories out. The "in" is through our mouths only. The "out" is via our engine—our metabolism. Our muscles, GI tract, and other "working parts."

To calculate the number of calories you burn every day, multiply your weight by 15 if moderately active, by 13 if you get little exercise, to get the approximate number of calories burned/day. This should be your intake if you wish to remain stable.

The "way of life" is that you become "more padded" during and after midlife. This certainly does not mean, however, that you have to gain 5-10 lbs. a year through your midlife passage. It does mean, however, that if you don't want to gain, you have to work at it. No free lunch (no pun intended). Specifically, what can you do?

1. Eat less. Drastically trimming calories is the only reliable way known to increase the life span of animals. Human animals are no different. Cutting portion size goes a huge way towards improving health.
2. Eat more often. Your digestive "engine" is a major source of calorie burning. If the engine works 4-5 times instead of 2-3 times each day, the resultant caloric loss is greater. This does not mean adding a couple of meals to what you already take in. Simply spread out the meals you normally eat into more "meals."

   For example: Drink your coffee and have your cereal at breakfast time, but reserve the fruit you would have put in the cereal and the muffin or toast for mid-morning. Have that salad and just a little of the bread for lunch, saving the rest of the bread and maybe the soup or the dessert for mid-afternoon; the fish and the broccoli for supper, leaving the beans or the pasta for a later snack. You get the picture.
3. Drink lots of water.
4. Work out! Exercise! Make sure you do some weights/weight-bearing work also so as to build up some muscle mass. Although muscle weighs more than fat, it sure looks and feels better and, even when you're not using it, metabolizes far more calories. Plus, muscle tissue takes up less

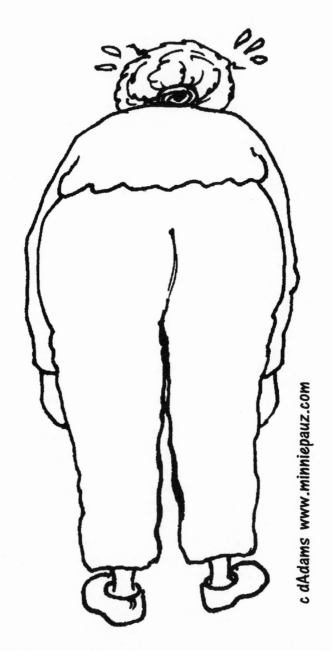

c dAdams www.minniepauz.com

# If God meant for me to touch my toes, he would have put them on my knees!

space than fat tissue for the same weight, so the more muscle you build up, the smaller your measurements will be. So keep that motor runnin'!

Also note that we tend to lose muscle and gain fat at and after midlife. As women age, they tend to redistribute their body fat to their abdomen ("apple shape"). Interestingly, estrogen supplementation/replacement therapy tends to maintain the traditional female fat distribution ("pear shape"). [All we need now is a pineapple and banana and we've got a fruit salad!]

## CANCER PREVENTION (see also Chapter 13)

Well, of course, genetics plays a part. That said, what can you do?

1. Think positively; be agreeable; diminish stress in your life; meditate. These all serve to boost your immune system.
2. Eat right! Along with thinking positively, this probably has the greatest effect on your ability to avoid cancer. I've already outlined what I mean: whole grains, good carbs, "fatty" fish, fresh fruits and veggies, nuts. Avoid fatty meats, fried foods, baked goods, processed and "fast foods."
3. Quit smoking; alcohol in moderation.
4. Avoid inhaled toxins from smoking or pollution.
5. Catch it early!
    a. Annual physical; Pap smear; mammograms
    b. Yearly ultrasound of the ovaries after age 40, if family history places you at risk or if your exam is difficult for your doctor (because of obesity, position of ovaries or if it's tough for you to relax).
    c. Annual check for "occult blood" in your stool; colonoscopy every 5 years if at risk, every 10 years if not. Who's at risk for colon cancer? Anyone with one first generation (mother, father, siblings) or two second generation relatives (aunt, grandfather, etc.) who has had colon cancer; anyone with a strong family history of breast and/or ovarian cancer; anyone with a long dietary history of lots of meats and fats and little fiber and fresh fruits and veggies.
    d  Have any abnormal bleeding, belly pain, abnormal lumps or growing dark skin moles investigated promptly.
    e. If you have a strong family history of breast cancer (2 first generation relatives), or a history of breast cancer and ovarian cancer and colon cancer, ask your health care practitioner to do a genetic analysis for "BrCa-I" and "BrCa-II" genes.

## HOW NOT TO DIE FROM A HEART ATTACK

Be alert to the warning signs of a heart attack. Prolonged chest pain or feeling of pressure is the most common symptom in men and women. Other symptoms include prolonged pain in the upper abdomen; pain from the chest to the left shoulder and arm, back, or jaw; shortness of breath, nausea or vomiting, and breaking out in a cold sweat.

If you suspect a heart attack, call 911 and your physician right away and then take an aspirin tablet. If you feel you may be going into "cardiac arrest" (severe suffocating chest pain, inability to catch your breath, feeling like you're about to pass out) take a very deep breath and initiate a series of as strong, severe, deep coughs as you can. The deep breath gets you oxygen and the severe coughs are about the best you can do to approximate the "chest compressions" given by cardiac resuscitation.

It may save your life some day.

## BEV'S STORY

Bev Sykes is my office manager. When I hired her a year and a half ago, I was, of course, aware that she was large, although I wasn't aware of her exact weight. In my office, where I emphasize health, exercise, and nutrition, I would have liked to have had someone a little more svelte, but Bev had the credentials and a bit of a warped sense of humor that I felt would fit right in. Plus, she appeared to be able to tolerate my craziness. She was hired!

I never once commented on Bev's weight, although I did ask if she might change the blue glasses with the little bunnies imbedded in the frame. Since she was a person who had successfully raised five children, born in the span of 6 years, I gave her some leeway, understanding the mental health stresses of that experience.

We got along well. Patients came and went by Bev's desk, frequently leaving to the strains of "...and don't forget to exercise" and "...you don't have to like it, you just have to do it." One day, along about last March, I looked at Bev and realized, "You've lost some weight."

"Thirteen pounds, to be exact," Bev replied exultantly. It was then that Bev told me of her "program."

Bev is 60 (or as she likes to remind me, "2 weeks older than you are: just remember that.") She hadn't had a physical exam in several years. At her exam in January, she discovered that she was hypertensive (155/100), had diabetes (her fasting blood sugar was 180 and her hemoglobin A1C almost 7), and had a cholesterol level of 215 with low HDLs–a bad combination. She had "weighed in" at 315 lbs! Her body mass index was somewhere over 45.

"After I was diagnosed with the diabetes, I realized that I was putting my health in danger. There were just too many things I wanted to stay around and do. Previously, every time I dieted it was to lose weight and it always came back. This time it was to get healthy!"

Bev had literally never exercised in her life. She joined Weight Watchers™ and was attending a meeting at 8:30 every Tuesday morning. She was following a "dietary exchange" plan outlined by Weight Watchers which emphasized good nutrition and calorie control.

Equally importantly, she had started to exercise. She discovered the joys of bike riding (after all, we live in Davis, California, which has more bicycles per capita than any other city in the USA. Here it is considered poor form not to own a bike.) She was riding a half hour every morning and that day in fact, she had for the first time biked the five miles to work. She had started to go on weekend "excursions" and was going riding that weekend with a friend of hers in Berkeley. And she joined "Curves™."

"For the first two weeks I was sore in muscles I didn't know existed," Bev told me, "but now that I've been riding three weeks, I feel much better. I wasn't able to ride yesterday and I missed it!"

Bev's twice monthly adventures have now grown to 20-30+ miles. She still rides daily. Although she "fell off the wagon" and gained several pounds over Christmas, she is now down to 230 lbs. (85 lbs. off over 11 months!) She had no poundage goal when she started ("just to get healthy") and she still doesn't, although I know she'd like to get down to or below 200 lbs.

And, although she still had to go on a mild antihypertensive, her blood sugars have reverted to normal and she's avoided diabetic medication! Her cholesterol? Down to 145!

Bev tells me that she keeps her old clothes in the closet "to remind myself." She's buying new clothing sparingly, awaiting weight stability before obtaining a new wardrobe. I'm sure spending all that money on new clothes will help prevent relapse.

She is still no easier to live with, though. And Monday she again wore the blue glasses!

*It's never too late to have a fling*
*for autumn is just as nice as spring*
*and it's never too late to fall in love.*
                          —Sandy Wilson, *The Boyfriend*

# CHAPTER TWELVE

## MENOPAUSE AND AFTER
"Do I have to be on this stuff forever??"

...It's really up to you.

Nowadays, a woman on hormonal supplementation must feel a little like a Christian Scientist with appendicitis. Used to be that when a woman asked her doc, "How long do I have to be on these hormones?" the answer was either "forever" or, tongue in cheek, "only until you're 90."

Now, in one of those 180 degree medical flip-flops, we're told "well, maybe you shouldn't take it at all...and if you do, only for a short period of time."

We've talked about this several times earlier and I think you know my general feeling: dosage no higher than needed, time not longer than necessary. What, then, is the case for "hormones forever"?

It boils down, I guess, to how you feel "on" hormones and how you feel "off." We've spoken several times about how and when to "taper down." What if each time you try to taper off, you just don't feel as well, or have symptoms that don't go away and aren't corrected by any of the pills and potions given by your physician, nurse practitioner, or herbalist. What, specifically, are the risks if you "want to be on the stuff forever"?

There's an increase of approximately 7-8 cases per 10,000 women per year of thromboembolism (blood clots which could travel to your brain or lungs), gall stones, breast cancer (probably not evident until after 4/5 years on hormones). These risks may be much lower for low-dose estrogens.

Speaking plainly, that means an additional risk of 70-80 cases per 10,000 (or 7-8 per 1,000) of these maladies after 10 years, or approximately 150 per 10,000 (15 per 1,000 or 1.5 per 100) after 20 years.

Cardiovascular-wise, the increased risk of a major "event" on HRT comes in the first year or two on supplementation; after that time, hormones are at least neutral and probably heart-healthy.

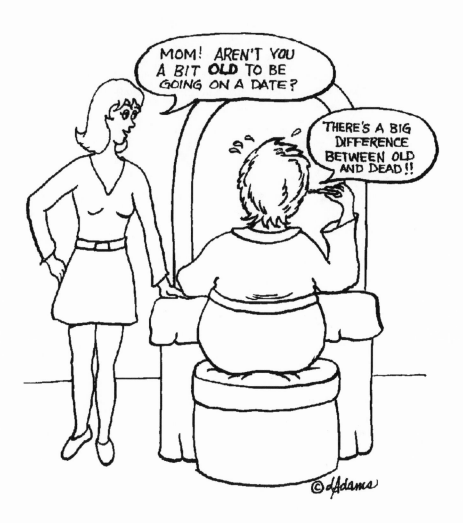

Likewise, hormones help prevent osteoporosis (as do several other things), and help prevent colon cancer (by about the same percentage: 7-8 cases per 10,000 women per year).

Armed with this information, you can make an informed decision. Exactly how much better do you feel on estrogens that you feel these risks are worth it for day-by-day better quality of life? Or, conversely, do you really feel that much worse when off estrogens?

There is no indication of any long term negative consequences from isoflavones or botanicals. But, at the same time, so far there have been no long term studies that would tell if there were any long term risks (besides, they cost a lot!). *Caveat emptor.*

Likewise, regarding testosterone. There are no long term studies to guide us. (Although there are a lot of older men around, they don't live to be as old as women, do they? And if they do, is it related to testosterone levels?)

Certainly, if you elect to continue on HRT well past menopause, I'd consider the lowest dose the safest and make efforts periodically to taper off.

And remember: if your rationale for long-term estrogen usage revolves around preserving and helping to correct your bone density, a SERM will do this just as well as estrogen without some of estrogen's added risks (although SERMs also have an added risk of thromboembolism—blood clots—similar to estrogens).

Likewise, although long term estrogens can help with your lipid profile, statins do this better and have a very favorable risk profile (and may help preserve bone density at the same time).

*I am worn to a raveling*
—Beatrix Potter

*There's nothing on my mind that couldn't be expressed by a long insane burst of hysterical rage.*
—Ashley Brilliant

# CHAPTER THIRTEEN

## THE STRESS CONNECTION
### Immunologic Health and the Placebo Effect; How Stress Affects Everything—and What To Do

It's amazing how intricately stress is involved in the moment-to-moment issues of comfort and discomfort, health and disease in our lives, and how little we really do know about it (other than to acknowledge its presence).

We are all "stressed out" about something or other, but we rarely do more than complain about how stressed out we are.

"Stress" is when you're nervous about something. Anxious. Not at ease. When you're "angst-ing" over something. When you're doing something and worried that you're not doing enough.

Stress has always been a component of life, but in "modern high-pressure existence" and certainly during mid-life and the peri-menopausal years, other factors are afoot to exacerbate the situation.

The CAUSES OF STRESS for midlife women are multiple:

One's body and body image are changing-omnipresent weight issues are frequently magnified (an apt choice of words, unfortunately).

Our children are frequently teenagers. Or they're leaving the home and the resultant echoes are haunting. Or else we're left to care for their children (our grandchildren) as our children's lives crumble around them. (Parenthood forever!) Stress.

Frequently we have our own aging parents to care for, and life comes full circle as we become the caregivers of our previous caregivers. Stress.

The economy and job market are changing. Previously secure jobs and financial footings become shaky and less secure. The pressures of both our jobs and those of our mate are frequently accentuated. Stress.

Sexual and personal tensions may build between ourselves and the mate who may now seem more distant or unavailable. If our sexual desire has waned, an additional edginess enters our relationship. Stress.

For these and other reasons, we may become depressed. We are certainly more aware of health issues and our own mortality as for the first time we are told of our high blood pressure, or irregular heartbeat. As we have our first colonoscopy. When our best friend or next door neighbor gets breast cancer. More stress.

This STRESS IMPACTS OUR HEALTH in many ways, the link most likely being the Immune System.

Why do some people get colds when a child coughs across the street, while another can be on a crowded subway during flu season and come through unscathed? The Immune System.

Why do some people get herpes once and then never again and some have monthly recurrences? The Immune System.

Why do some people with AIDS survive for years and years while some go rapidly downhill? The Immune System.

Why are some people sick all the time, and others are not? You guessed it: the Immune System.

But stress adversely impacts health in other ways too. Highly stressed individuals (including so-called Type A Personalities) have a far greater rate of cardiovascular disease. (In fact, highly-stressed individuals should have closer monitoring of their C-reactive protein and homocysteine levels as indicators of risk for cardiovascular disease.)

It is well known that stress leads to (or certainly exacerbates) irritable bowel syndrome and other gastrointestinal maladies.

Stress produces sleep difficulties (insomnia) in many individuals, which then leads to lessened productivity, more mood disturbances, and less resistance to infection, etc.

And what about cancer?? It is not unreasonable to hypothesize that increased levels of stress lead to a greater incidence of all types of cancer. (I'll bet at a far greater level than the "7-8 more cases of breast cancer per 10,000 women per year" that has so many women and their physicians freaked out about HRT!)

There is no meaningful data on the relationship of stress to cancer. But why do some people survive (or at least last longer) with different types of cancer, and some go so rapidly downhill?

Back to our old friend the Immune System. Stress weakens it; calm and positive thinking enhances it. It's that simple.

## COPING WITH STRESS

Many full-length books have been written on this subject alone and I shall not attempt to compete. I'll simply outline and describe the things (and tricks) I work with in my practice.

They work. You really have no choice: stay stressed (and sleep poorly and expose yourself to a much greater risk of bad diseases) or WORK ON IT.

C'mon: You can do it!!

Trim activities from your daily list. Start out by dropping one thing per day from your list. (Absolutely no new substitutions for the dropped activity!).

Have someone else do the dropped activity! Spouse, offspring, employee, etc. Delegate responsibility.

I know: no one can do it as good as you. But that's your choice to make. You can't lose stress if you take it all on. Can you realize that, yes, it may be done differently? Maybe better; probably in your eyes, worse. That is the trade you must make if you are to lessen your stress. It's a tough one, but a necessary trade.

## RELAXATION SKILLS:

### Meditation.

If you are to settle yourself, you must, regularly, cleanse your mind. That's what meditation is all about: cleansing one's mind of all the clitter-clatter, worries, angers, anticipations and concerns that bug us, stress us, and hazard our sleep.

What is meditation? Anything that makes it difficult or impossible to THINK while you are doing the activity. Vigorous exercise is a meditation (it's hard to worry about a project or anger directed toward a neighbor while you're puffing on the treadmill set at 4 with a 5% grade!).

Yoga is a meditation. There are many meditation techniques and they all work the same: to cleanse the mind for a period of time. (It's hard to be thinking while you're practicing paced respiration, body awareness, "Ommming" or chanting a mantra over and over again to yourself.)

My favorite meditation (which is nice because you can do it anywhere and even 10 minutes helps) is a breath meditation (called Anapana Breathing, a form of Samatha meditation), or a whole body sensory awareness (Vipassana meditation).

Here's how it works: Anapana Breathing is best done for 15-30 minutes at the beginning and the end of each day. Find a quiet, comfortable area where you can sit cross-legged with pillows supporting your back (and knees, if needed), as free of stimulation (lights, kids, TV, telephone, pets, etc.) as possible. With arms comfortably on your legs, close your eyes and concentrate on slow deep breaths, in and out through your nose. Concentrate only on the touch of the breaths, in and out, on your upper lip, nose, nostrils, windpipe, filling your lungs-cooler air coming in; warmer going out. Maybe through one nostril, maybe both. As you go in and out, remain quiet, accepting, "equanamous." You are steady. You are a rock. You are still water. If "thoughts" enter your head, chase them away with breathing and concentration.

You may feel sensations (prickles, cramps, twinges) in other parts of your body: acknowledge them, but always return to the breathing. Concentrate on the touch of the breath and on the continual changing sensations in the body and remain equanamous, in the present moment.

"Fine Tuning." Identify the in breath as the "in breath," and the out breath as the "out breath." Pay attention only to the touch of the breath. Stop thinking. Be aware. Breathe in: calm the body. Breathe out: smile. Be in the present moment.

You can, if you wish, add visualization (a la Thich Nhat Hanh, a Vietnamese Buddhist master) to your meditation.

Some exercises are

| Breathe in—I see myself as | Breathe out—I feel: |
|---|---|
| A flower | Fresh |
| A mountain | Solid |
| Still water | Calm and still |
| Open space | Free |
| Alive | Mindful (I smile to myself) |

If you have mastered Samattha meditation, you may go deeper to Vipassana meditation. In brief, this is extending concentration on the breath to a slow assessment of any and all sensations (tingling, tightening, twitching, itching, cramping, crawling, etc., etc.) on the skin or deeper, starting at the top of the scalp and going down to your toes and up again, down again, etc., surveying all parts of your body. No judgment, no "feeling good" or "feeling bad." Remaining equanamous and realizing that every one of these sensations rises up, and passes away. Changing, changing–always changing.

And, before you know it, 15 or 30 or more minutes have passed away. Always end your meditation with good thoughts of your family or friends or whomever. ("May all beings be happy.")

You will be refreshed and function better. Sleep better also.

(For further information access http://www.mahavana.dhama.org, or check out Vipassana on any good search engine.)

Roll Breathing.

Another take on breath meditation is Roll Breathing. The object is to develop full use of your lungs and get in touch with the rhythm of your breathing. To do this, place your left hand on your abdomen and your right hand on your chest. Notice how your hands move as you breathe in and out. Practice filling your lower lungs by breathing so that your left hand goes up when you inhale while your right hand remains still. Inhale through your nose, exhale through your mouth.

When you've filled and emptied your lower lungs 8-10 times with ease, add this second step: inhale first into your lower lungs as before, but continue inhaling into your upper chest. As you do this, your right hand will rise and your left hand fall, as your chest fills.

As you exhale slowly through your mouth, make a quiet "whooshing" sound as first your left hand and then your right hand fall. As you exhale, feel tension leave your body as you become more and more relaxed.

Practice breathing in and out this way for 5 minutes or so and notice that the movement of your abdomen and chest is like rolling waves, rising and falling in rhythmic motions. This technique should be practiced daily for several weeks until (like Anapana Breathing) it can be done almost everywhere, providing you with an instant relaxation tool any time you need it.

## Progressive Muscle Relaxation

The body responds to tense thoughts or situations with muscle tension, which can cause pain or discomfort. Deep muscle relaxation reduces the muscle tension as well as general mental anxiety. You can go through all the muscle groups by just tensing and relaxing each one. Deep muscle relaxation is effective in combating stress-related health problems and often helps you get to sleep.

To practice this procedure, pick a place where you can stretch out comfortably, such as a carpeted floor. Tense each muscle group for 4-10 seconds (hard, but not to the point of cramping) and then give yourself 10-20 seconds to release and relax. At various points, review the various muscle groups and relax each one a little more each time.

Examples of how to tense muscle groups follow:

1. Hands by clenching them.
2. Wrists and forearms by extending them and bending the hands back at the wrist.
3. Biceps and upper arms by clenching your hands into fists, bending your arms at the elbow and flexing your biceps.
4. Shoulders by shrugging them.
5. Forehead by wrinkling into a deep frown.
6. Around the eyes and bridge of the nose by closing the eyes as tightly as possible.
7. Cheeks and jaws by grinning from ear to ear.

8.  Around the mouth by pressing the lips tightly together.
9.  Back of the neck by pressing the head back hard.
10. Front of the neck by touching chin to the chest.
11. Chest by taking a deep breath and holding it, then exhaling.
12. Back by arching the back up and away from the floor.
13. Stomach by sucking it into a hard knot.
14. Hips and buttocks by pressing the buttocks tightly together.
15. Thighs by clenching them hard.
16. Lower legs by pointing the toes toward the face as if trying to bring the toes up to touch the head.
17. Lower legs by pointing the toes away and curling the toes downward at the same time.

These tensions may be done all together from top to bottom, or working on specific muscle groups at one time. When you are finished, arouse yourself thoroughly by counting backwards from 5 to 1.

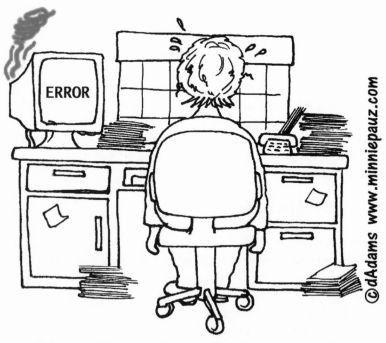

**Ok Lord, it's Monday....if I have even one tiny hormone left in my body....GIVE IT TO ME NOW!**

Relaxation Response

The relaxation response is the exact opposite of a stress response. It slows heart rate and helps breathing, lowers blood pressure and helps relieve muscle tension. The technique (adapted from Herbert Benson, M.D.), is:

1. Sit quietly in a comfortable position with eyes closed.
2. Begin progressive muscle relaxation
3. Become aware of your breathing. With each exhale say the word "one" (or any other word or phrase) silently or aloud. Concentrate on breathing from your abdomen and not your chest. Instead of focusing on a repeated word, you may choose to fix your gaze on a stationary object (you may set up a little altar, if you wish). Any mental stimulus will help you shift your mind away from external thoughts.
4. Continue this for 10-20 minutes. As distracting thoughts enter your mind, don't dwell on them, just allow them to drift away.
5. Sit quietly for several minutes, until you are ready to open your eyes.
6. Notice the difference in your breathing and your pulse rate.

Don't worry whether you are successful in becoming deeply relaxed. The key is to remain impassive. To let distracting thoughts slip away like waves on the beach.

Practice for 10-30 minutes once or twice a day, but not within 2 hours after a meal. When you've set up a routine, the relaxation response should come with little effort.

It makes absolutely no difference which method(s) you choose. Feel free to "mix and match," to devise your own personal method. The important thing is to do it ideally at the beginning and the end of each day. Promise you'll give yourself a 2-week trial. See how you feel!

**Other Advice Regarding Stress Relaxation:**

Be active! There's nothing like a brisk walk or visit to the health club to chase away tension.

Aging parents can certainly be a cause of stress. Do not feel that you must take on the entire responsibility by yourself. Look actively into community support programs (you'd be surprised what is available in most communities)-check your local Senior Center or service clubs.

Whatever it is, you do not have to do it alone. Get help!

This includes counseling. As indicated in previous chapters, therapists of differing sex and therapeutic orientation are available to help. Also, many communities have yoga centers, stress reduction counselors, meditation teachers, and other mentors available.

Don't say "...I don't have enough time." That's just admitting that stress and your sources of stress are more important than your health and peace of mind.

### The Placebo Effect and The Immune System
We've all heard of "placebos" and "the placebo effect" which somehow have negative connotations. Au contraire! The placebo effect is one of the most wonderful (and safest) results of many medical and paramedical therapies.

### Placebo is good.
What is placebo effect? It is that positive effect from a drug or treatment modality which does not stem from the active ingredient or supposed medicinal quality or qualities specifically attributed to that therapy. In other words, it is that positive effect that happens simply because we think it will help. Because we believe. In medical research, in order to find out if a given medication or treatment modality works, its benefits are compared to results from one which looks/feels/appears the same as the thing being tested, but which actually contains no active ingredient. To be judged effective, the actual drug or treatment must show a meaningful improvement ("statistically significant") over and above the sham drug or treatment.

For example, recently a new migraine medication (Maxalt®) was tested, pairing it against Imitrex® (considered the "gold standard" of migraine medications) and a placebo.

Headaches were "cured" in 30-35% of patients taking placebo, and 60-65% of patients taking the two medications, a statistically significant percentage. The new medication (Maxalt®) worked, as did the Imitrex®.

But what about the ⅓ of patients whose migraine was relieved by the little pill that contained no active ingredient? What are they? Chopped liver? No! They got better because they believed that that little bitty pill they swallowed would do something and that belief helped them (and with no medication side effects).

Is that bad?? Of course not!!

But how does it work, this placebo effect? How does someone heal, get better, stave off cancer, live for 10 years when only given 6 months.

The "power of positive thinking." (Thank you, Norman Vincent Peale!) Of believing. The power of Lourdes. The power of meditation.

Most likely, the placebo effects from simple relief of headache to miraculous cancer cures have to do with the strengthening of one's own bodily defenses, one's Immune System, resulting from the mind-body interaction called in to play.

The Immune System, one's innate army to do battle with disease can be either little more than a ragtag, ill-equipped band of peasants, or a mightily armored fortress. Genetics plays a part, but certainly so does the psyche. The belief. The positive feelings that translate to a physical, physiological, and biological improvement of one's own immune potential.

### Stress and "Adrenal Fatigue"

This is controversial and not proven with large peer-review studies. But it makes clinical and common sense.

Just as Insulin Resistance (where the body is resistant to the effects of its own insulin and the pancreas has to work overtime) increases the risk of diabetes it is felt that chronic stress, chronic "fight or flight" statically increases the adrenals' output. They must continually work. Frequently in these women, the blood or salivary cortisol (an adrenal hormone) is normal or elevated, as are DHEA and pregnenalone (although not infrequently serum pregnenalone is on the low side). The adrenal gland is "pushing" to maintain homeostasis, but there is little reserve.

## RENATE'S STORY

Renate Holcomb came into my office accompanied by her husband (to make sure she actually kept her appointment, I think; once she was actually here, he took off shopping for awhile).

As we began our interview, Renate told me, "I guess you'd call me a 'cranky person,' but recently-especially the last 2-3 months-I've been especially cranky and tired. Frank (her husband) is used to me, but now I'm even on his nerves."

Renate had been on HRT with PremPro®, which she had discontinued 3 months previously, but the "cranky and tired" symptoms had antedated her stopping HRT. Because of problems with insomnia, she had restarted her hormone pills about 6-8 weeks ago; the insomnia was a little better since that time, but the crankiness and tiredness remained.

Additionally, Renate told me that she was "miserable" because of chronic back spasms which she'd had for several years, but was noticeably worse over the past 6 months.

"I want someone else's opinion," she told me, "regarding my risks of breast cancer, being on hormone therapy." One of her sisters developed breast cancer at age 42; her other sister was on tamoxifen because of the family history plus the fact that she had "some calcifications that were being watched" and had had several breast biopsies.

"Mostly, though, I'd like to see why I'm so tired all the time!"

Additionally, Renate complained of vaginal dryness and was noting an almost daily very light vaginal spotting over the past year. She also noted that when she had temporarily stopped HRT, the bleeding had stopped entirely.

Her past history included sleep apnea. She was on two other medications, Wellbutrin® and Trazodone® (for depression and attention deficit hyperactivity disorder-ADHD) and recently had been started on Concerta® (long-acting Ritalin®) for the ADHD, and this more or less coincided with the onset of her insomnia problems.

Renate told me that she worked as an Internal Affairs Investigator, investigating employee misconduct in the State Department of Managed Care. "It's a high stress job," she told me, and I noticed for the first time a facial tic, sort of a tightening and twitching of her jaw muscles, that I was to see more of in time to come.

Her marital relationship was "mediocre," also with a lot of stress. As if that wasn't enough, lovemaking had recently become uncomfortable because of vaginal dryness. She was also having a bit of a problem with some urinary incontinence, but we decided to put that on the "back burner" for later.

I ordered several tests (thyroid, stool samples for occult blood, lipids, C-reactive protein and homocysteine, plus salivary testosterone, mammography and a peripheral bone density) and asked Renate to return the next week for an ultrasound to evaluate the cause of her bleeding. She was firmly advised to see an orthopedist and to do all possible to deal with her back problem, which I felt played a great part in her crankiness and fatigue.

Ultrasound a week later showed an approximately $\frac{3}{8}$ x $\frac{3}{8}$ x $\frac{3}{4}$ inch "density" in the uterus, consistent with an endometrial polyp, and this was confirmed when I put a little fluid into the uterus to "outline" it. A biopsy did not show any features of malignancy (the biopsy instrument actually slid off the polyp, which is quite difficult to sample), and I scheduled her for hysteroscopy to remove the polyp.

Renate informed me that she had stopped the Concerta® and her sleep had perhaps slightly improved. We spent some time in discussing a treatment protocol for her other issues. We decided to change HRT from Premarin® to transdermal estrogen (easier to down-regulate) and from Provera® to Prometrium® ("gentler" on the system, and, when taken at bedtime, possibly leading to calmer, better sleep).

An exercise program was firmly outlined and strongly recommended, including 2-3 half hour sessions after work for weekdays and 2-hour-plus sessions on weekends. She was to cut her caffeine in half and work her way down from there. Her labs were all OK, although the salivary testosterone and DHEA were not back yet.

Renate returned and we discussed her probable endometrial polyp. She wished to delay her surgery "until after Christmas," 6 weeks away, and I concurred. We spent almost 45 minutes discussing her progress and new programs: she had cut down her previous "4-5 cups" of coffee to 2 cups per day.

She had not yet started to exercise. "I just can't seem to get off the dime," she told me. Although she intellectually understood the importance of exercise, she was having difficulty in actualizing this.

I told Renate that her testosterone was significantly lowered (15.8), although her DHEA was within the normal range (as it usually is).

I had Renate fill out both an SDS (a Self-Rating Depression Questionnaire) (Fig. 13-1) and a MENSI, to track the progress of her symptoms. The remainder of the time was spent in discussing a "bedtime ritual" (see next chapter) and stress reduction, and some "handouts" to that effect were given to her. She was started on testosterone lotion and on a low dose of DHEA (considered by some to be a testosterone enhancing hormone) for placebo reasons as much as anything.

At her return a month later, Renate told me, "I'm still not as enthusiastic as I'd like to be; I'm just kinda "going along"—not real perky, but definitely not as cranky."

I wasn't sure whether this involved discontinuing the Concerta®, switching her progestin to Prometrium® and estrogen to estradiol, cutting down on caffeine, or exercising–probably a combination of all of the above. "I have started to exercise," she confided, "but I sure don't like it." (I gave her my spiel about not having to like it, just having to do it.) She was doing some stress reduction work, but definitely not to the degree that she should be.

Her SDS (see Fig. 13-1) showed an index of 59, consistent with mild-moderate depression. I advised her to speak with her therapist about a possible medication change, perhaps adding in some Neurontin®.

Renate's surgery (hysteroscopy and polypectomy) took place uneventfully the day after Christmas. The pathology report was benign.

While we were actively focused on the workup and therapy of her bleeding, Renate seemed to be a bit more focused and at ease. However, when I saw her back for her post-op check a month later, her "twitch" was worse than ever. She had discontinued the DHEA as it "made me jittery." Her testosterone levels were a bit high and I adjusted her dosage downward. Her problems again were the same: insomnia and stress. In addition, her neck pain was worse than ever. She was exercising (but not enough) and was not really doing any stress reduction work. She had stopped bleeding, however.

# ZUNG SELF-RATING DEPRESSION SCALE (SDS)[5]

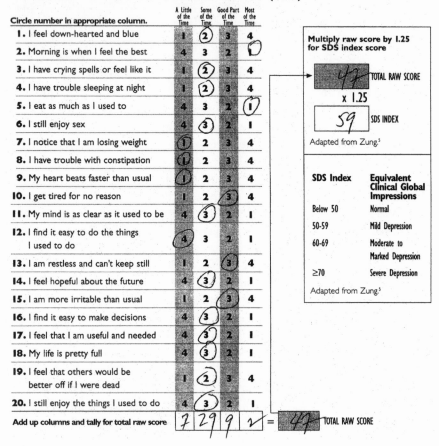

| Circle number in appropriate column. | A Little of the Time | Some of the Time | Good Part of the Time | Most of the Time |
|---|---|---|---|---|
| 1. I feel down-hearted and blue | 1 | (2) | 3 | 4 |
| 2. Morning is when I feel the best | 4 | 3 | 2 | (1) |
| 3. I have crying spells or feel like it | 1 | (2) | 3 | 4 |
| 4. I have trouble sleeping at night | 1 | (2) | 3 | 4 |
| 5. I eat as much as I used to | 4 | 3 | 2 | (1) |
| 6. I still enjoy sex | 4 | (3) | 2 | 1 |
| 7. I notice that I am losing weight | (1) | 2 | 3 | 4 |
| 8. I have trouble with constipation | (1) | 2 | 3 | 4 |
| 9. My heart beats faster than usual | (1) | 2 | 3 | 4 |
| 10. I get tired for no reason | 1 | 2 | (3) | 4 |
| 11. My mind is as clear as it used to be | 4 | (3) | 2 | 1 |
| 12. I find it easy to do the things I used to do | (4) | 3 | 2 | 1 |
| 13. I am restless and can't keep still | 1 | 2 | (3) | 4 |
| 14. I feel hopeful about the future | 4 | (3) | 2 | 1 |
| 15. I am more irritable than usual | 1 | 2 | (3) | 4 |
| 16. I find it easy to make decisions | 4 | (3) | 2 | 1 |
| 17. I feel that I am useful and needed | 4 | (3) | 2 | 1 |
| 18. My life is pretty full | 4 | (3) | 2 | 1 |
| 19. I feel that others would be better off if I were dead | 1 | (2) | 3 | 4 |
| 20. I still enjoy the things I used to do | 4 | (3) | 2 | 1 |
| Add up columns and tally for total raw score | 7 | 29 | 9 | 1 | = 47 TOTAL RAW SCORE |

Multiply raw score by 1.25
for SDS index score

47 TOTAL RAW SCORE

x 1.25

59 SDS INDEX

Adapted from Zung.[5]

| SDS Index | Equivalent Clinical Global Impressions |
|---|---|
| Below 50 | Normal |
| 50-59 | Mild Depression |
| 60-69 | Moderate to Marked Depression |
| ≥70 | Severe Depression |

Adapted from Zung.[5]

Figure 13-1. Zung Self-Rating Depression Scale*
*Zung, W.N.K., "A Self-Rating Depression Scale." Archives of Clinical Psychiatry, 1965, Vol. 12, pgs 63-70.

I made a direct referral to a good pain management anesthesia group, and we again discussed both a "bedtime ritual" and specific stress reduction routines. I gave Renate the name of a local couple who specialized in stress reduction techniques (although she told me she wasn't certain she would find the time to take advantage of this).

We started on a gentle taper-down schedule of her HRT, with plans to be at the lowest dose, and hopefully off altogether within a year, and we discussed the possibility (for breast cancer reduction and bone support) of starting her on raloxifene when the HRT was down.

I discussed also the (controversial) aspect of "adrenal fatigue" with Renate. Her serum pregnenalone was a bit low and, when repeated, low-normal. We talked pros and cons and decided on a low dose (50 mg) of transdermal pregnenalone, compounded together with her testosterone.

Renate is good at keeping her follow-up appointments (better than she is in actualizing therapy). I'm not sure she is capable of "lightening up," prioritizing what are the most important jobs and increasing peace of mind. Hopefully, between getting rid of some of her stressors (the vaginal bleeding, the insomnia and perhaps the neck pain), and an adjustment of her psych medications, she will be less fatigued and stressed. I hope she will continue exercising and truly try the stress reduction path.

Only time will tell.

*Sleep is when all the unsorted stuff comes flying out as from a dustbin upset in a high wind.*

—William Golding, *Pincher Martin*

# CHAPTER FOURTEEN

## INSOMNIA

What good are you if you can't sleep?

Certainly there is a wide range of "normality" in sleep requirements. Although my aunt may have gotten along on four hours of sleep a night, and my wife requires twelve, most people fall into the 6-10 hour range.

Normality aside, many midlife women suffer from sleep disturbances not present prior to their peri-menopausal years. Certainly, insomnia is one of the common and more disturbing symptoms of the peri-menopause and early menopausal years.

Sleep difficulties may be categorized into two types: difficulty in falling asleep and difficulty in staying asleep. During peri-menopause and post-menopause, both types can occur.

### Sleep Physiology

What happens during sleep? What produces a restful night's repose?

Without going into detail, there are different stages the pre-somnolent individual passes through on her way to dreamland. The normal person will pass up and down through the different layers of sleep several times each night. The deepest and most restful is dream sleep and is called REM sleep (for Rapid Eye Movement, which is what happens during dream sleep). The more REM sleep, the more restful your sleeping time will be.

Anything which serves to lighten sleep (like a hot flash or disturbing thoughts just underneath the veneer of your sleep) will both prevent REM sleep and tend to awaken you during the lighter phases of your sleep cycle.

Sleep Studies:

Many medical centers have Sleep Labs or Sleep Disorder Clinics that are specifically for the study of individuals with a sleep disorder (or chronic insomnia).

A "sleep study," or "nocturnal polysomnogram," as it is medically known, utilizes eye movement monitors, central and occipital (back of head) EEG, nasal and oral air flow monitors, chin and lower leg EMG (muscle movement) monitors, chest and abdominal excursion (breathing movement) monitors, EKG and pulse oximetry (measuring oxygen content of the blood).

These studies measure sleep architecture (stages of sleep, amount of REM sleep, numbers of "arousals," episodes of upper airway resistance (sleep apnea), leg movements, and EKG or EEG abnormalities).

If your insomnia is long-standing (antedating midlife changes) or does not improve with hormonal therapy or therapy of an underlying medical problem, changing medications, etc., a "sleep study" is a good idea. Ask your health care practitioner or local neurologist about this.

## What Causes Insomnia?

1. Negative life experiences.

A stressful life (family or workplace) or childhood or marital abuse can cause insomnia. Stress, anxiety and unresolved issues inhibit restful sleep by causing the brain to remain "on guard," producing what meditators refer to as "monkey mind." A "chattering mind," worrying and thinking-thinking-thinking impedes the fog of sleep from settling in and, during those nocturnal times during which one gets "light" (out of deep REM sleep), the chatter awakens the poor "monkey."

2. Medical Problems

"Restless leg syndrome" (and its milder cousin, "periodic limb movements") may cause leg pain or discomfort at night.

Sleep apnea is a condition in which breathing periodically stops— sometimes hundreds of time each night. The "survival centers" in the brain, recognizing the lack of oxygen, partially awaken the individual, who resumes breathing. Frequently this is caused by the uvula (the little flap of skin beyond your tongue) falling against the windpipe (called "obstructive sleep apnea") which also produces snoring.

Restless leg syndrome is usually treated with medications, vitamins and other preventive measures. Sleep apnea may require surgery, special respiratory devices (called C-PAP which "forces" a breath promptly without awakening the individual), or occasionally surgery to shorten the uvula in cases of obstructive sleep apnea. Periodic limb movements or restless leg syndrome are frequently one of the insomnia components of peri-menopausal women and usually respond promptly to estrogen replacement therapy.

Significant anemia can also predispose to poor quality sleep. A "hemogram" or "CBC" (complete blood count) should be performed and can help rule out anemia.

3.   Menopause

The hormonal changes of menopause and the night sweats they produce can disrupt sleep.

It is not older age per se but the menopausal transition itself, independent of other factors, that is associated with sleep difficulties.

As women reach mid-life and enter the menopausal transition, rates of sleep difficulty increase dramatically. The steep hormonal ups and downs of the peri-menopause, and the later static "down" of the post-menopause affect the temperature regulatory centers of the brain, causing tiny nerves surrounding many small blood vessels to send out a signal which leads to dilatation or opening of these vessels, temporarily increasing blood flow to the skin, producing the "flash" or sweat.

Whereas insomnia is uncommon among persons younger than 20 years, approximately 20-25% of women and 14-15% of men report sleep difficulties between 45-49 years old, and 40% of women (but only 15% of men) in one large study[1] report not sleeping well by their early 50s. Caucasian and Hispanic women reported the highest rates of sleep difficulty. Japanese and Chinese reported the lowest, with African American women being intermediate.

The percentage of women experiencing sleep difficulties is highest in those who are in late menopause and in those with surgical menopause not receiving HRT.

Menopause affects sleep quality in ways other than through effects of hot flashes, including an increased prevalence of sleep apnea and especially periodic limb movement disorders. Additionally, the social changes of mid-age such as reentering the workforce, stress, aging and sometimes caring for older parents may have adverse effects.

4.   Disruption of the Body's Internal Clock

Some people have what is called the "advanced sleep phase syndrome," falling asleep very early in the evening and awakening very early in the morning. People with "delayed sleep phase syndrome" fall asleep very late and awaken late the following day.

5.   Lifestyle Factors

Intake of caffeine within 4-6 hours of bedtime, excessive alcohol consumption prior to sleep (2 or more drinks) and vigorous exercise near bedtime can all affect one's ability to get to sleep or stay asleep. Even small amounts of caffeine can disrupt sleep in sensitive individuals. Excess stress,

---

[1]"Sleep Difficulty in Women at Midlife: A Community Survey of Sleep and the Menopause Transition," by Ganz et al in <u>Menopause: The Journal of the No. Am. Menopause Society</u>, Vol. 10, #1, 2003

obviously, can both affect the ability to get to sleep or stay asleep during the "light times" of sleep's rhythm ("monkey mind").

6. Medications

A plethora of medications (some more than others) can interfere with sleep, especially in sensitive individuals. The list includes: antidepressants (especially Wellbutrin® and the SSRIs, Prozac®, Zoloft®, etc.);

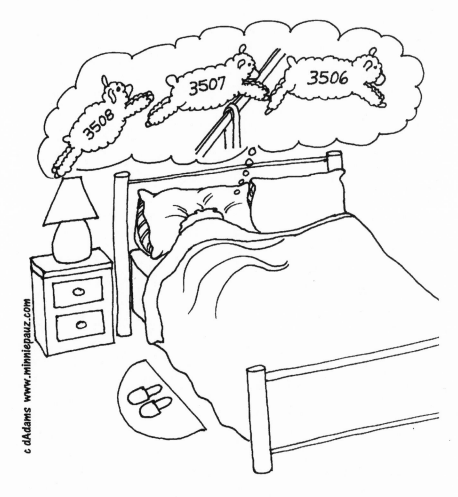

bronchodilators (asthma medications); beta blockers (a class of high blood pressure medications, including Tenormin®, Corgard®, Inderal®, Betapace®, etc.); central nervous system stimulants (amphetamines, appetite suppressants and other medications such as Cylert®, Concerta®, etc.); steroids (androgenic agents; glucocorticoids such as Decadron®, hydrocortisone, Medrol®, etc.); respiratory agents such as Aerobid®,

Azmacort®, Flovent®, QVar®, etc.; and decongestants containing pseudoephedrine (Sudafed®).

## Treatment Strategies

Insomnia caused by a medical problem or hormonal change usually clears up when the underlying condition is treated.

Therapy can be divided into several approaches. If you haven't gotten a good night's sleep in weeks, a short-acting sleeping pill (e.g. Ambien® or Sonata®) can be life-saving while you're starting "behavioral therapy" (see below) and/or hormonal or other therapy for peri-menopausal symptoms, if appropriate.

1.  Behavioral Therapies

Exercise for at least 30 minutes daily. Weight-lifting, aerobic workouts and other exercise may promote good sleep. But, don't exercise within 3 hours of bedtime. The best is outdoor morning exercise-exposure to light helps regulate the body clock (more about this later).

Avoid caffeine (coffee, cola, black/green tea, chocolate, "Excedrin®" or other headache medications with caffeine) after noon, especially within 6-8 hours of bedtime.

Try to go to bed and get up at the same time every day (including weekends). Avoid naps (even short ones) if you have trouble getting to sleep. (Naps make it harder to fall asleep at night.)

Don't drink alcohol at night. (Certainly not over 1 drink.) Alcohol makes sleep less restful. Also, avoid heavy meals late in the evening.

2.  Bedtime Ritual

A bedtime relaxation "ritual" can be very helpful enabling sleep. Additionally, an evening meditation can help clear the mind, promoting less awakening and more restful sleep. (If your mind is "chattering," you will not sleep as deeply and when you are "light," these "thoughts" are more likely to awaken you and make it more difficult to resume sleep.)

Relax an hour before bedtime. Read, listen to music, take a hot bath. Avoid activities that cause anxiety such as paying bills or watching the news!

I advise a "bedtime ritual" as follows:

a.  No stimulants at or after dinner, minimal alcohol with or after supper. No strenuous activities after supper.

b.  Draw a warm bath. Set candles around the tub (with soothing music, if available). Sip a mug of herbal tea/warm milk/hot water with lemon and honey, etc. and soak for 10-15 minutes.

c.  15-30 minutes of meditation before sleep.

3. Relieve peri-menopausal symptoms

   If awakening dripping with nighttime hot flashes and/or mood changes/irritability are part of your insomnia equation, of paramount importance is to promptly treat these symptoms. In this situation, short-term hormonal therapy starting with a mid-dose estrogen and then tapering down may be dramatically beneficial. Certainly an alternative may be therapy with progesterone cream, vitamin E, Effexor®, phytoestrogens and herbs. This may take longer, but it is certainly worth a try if you'd rather avoid estrogens (which you can always try if the non-hormonal methods are ineffective).

   Hot flashes and periodic limb movements are the peri-menopausal components of insomnia that respond well to hormonal supplementation, usually significantly improving quality sleep.

4. Light Therapy

   Increase daytime exposure to bright light with no exposure to bright light late in the day or evening.

   More specifically, you can sit in front of a "light box" or a bright light source for 30 minutes daily. Do this first thing in the morning if you have trouble falling asleep, and in the afternoon or evening if you wake up too early. Middle-of-the-night awakenings, however, usually aren't caused by body clock disturbances and aren't likely to respond to light therapy.

   (Light boxes and lamps that produce 10,000 lux—the recommended amount of light—are available from Light Therapy Products: (800) 426-6723; www.lighttherapyproducts.com)

5. Medications

   If you are at your wit's end because you haven't had a restful night sleep in weeks, there is nothing wrong with short-term drug therapy until the underlying cause of your insomnia is, hopefully, dealt with. These are divided into short-term and long-term medications.

   Short term (usually 2-3 weeks or less): The most commonly prescribed drugs for short-term use are zolpidem (Ambien®) and zaleplon (Sonata®). These are relatively safe and effective if taken under a physician's guidance and promote rapid relief for many insomniacs. Diminishing the fear of further sleeplessness can help break the cycle and escalation of insomnia.

   Ambien®, taken at bedtime, works for 7-8 hours; it helps people get to sleep and eliminates middle-of-the-night awakenings. Sonata® wears off in 4 hours. It can be taken at bedtime if you have trouble falling asleep or in the middle of the night if you awaken and can't get back to sleep (better than getting up, paying bills, or watching late night TV!).

Longer acting benzodiazepines, including Dalmane®, diazepam (Valium®), lorazepam (Ativan®), temazepam (Restoril®) are effective but may cause "daytime hangover effect." Others, including triazolam (Halcion®) cause less of a hangover effect, but if used on a prolonged basis may occasionally cause "rebound insomnia," which can be worse than the original insomnia.

Long term: The goal of the use of sleep medication for insomnia is as a short-term band-aid to "stop the bleeding," while the source is being treated.

However, in some individuals, insomnia is a chronic long-term proposition. Given the choice of taking medication long-term or being chronically insomniac, many persons will choose taking medications.

This obviously is a decision made between you and your physician and/or therapist.

Several medications are available to help you stay asleep, using these on a long term basis. These include Trazodone®, Halcion®, Restoril®, and others.

Over-the-counter agents that contain antihistamines such as diphenhydramine (Benadryl®, Tylenol P.M.®) and others (Unisom®, etc.) may work well for some individuals. The effects of these medications, however, are unpredictable. Some people don't get the sedation necessary for sleep; others experience next-day drowsiness.

Herbs and supplements: The herb valerian as a tablet, capsule, tincture or tea, taken an hour before bedtime may help, but its effectiveness is highly unpredictable, helping some, but not others. The usual dose is 300-600 mg of standardized extracts.

Kava has been used as a sleep aid and anti-anxiety medication. Its effect also is unpredictable and has been linked to liver damage if used chronically. I would recommend liver testing for women using Kava on a long-term basis.

Melatonin may be helpful for temporary "time clock readjustment" (e.g., long distance flights, radical changes in work schedule). Its long-term use is ill-advised and has been linked indirectly to infertility and heart disease.

6. Therapy for Obstructive Sleep Disorders (e.g., sleep apnea)

The "assisted breathing" available with a C-PAP unit prevents, in many individuals, the frequent "mini-awakenings" associated with obstructed air flow. In some individuals, however, this may be so severe as to require a surgical reduction in the size of their uvula. If this is your situation, make sure to discuss this with either a sleep physiologist, neurologist, or ENT specialist.

# MALINDA'S STORY

Mary Malinda Hart is my wife, so I'm pretty close to this one. She said I could tell her story if I bought her a 3-carat diamond ring, so I hope a lot of people buy this book, or I'm in deep trouble!

Malinda has always required a lot of sleep. As far back as she can remember, she's needed 10-12 hours at night or she does not feel rested (translation: grouchy) the next day. Even with this, she can nap if given the opportunity.

She is also the world's lightest sleeper—there's no sneaking into bed with Malinda—a deep sigh will wake her up. This, combined with a relatively small bladder, does not lead to productive, restful, high-REM sleep. When she is up, however, she's a dynamo. The dynamism was tempered a bit by the several years of "somnolence interruptus" following the birth of our son. Malinda still managed, however, with daytime naps supplementing her fragmented nighttime sleep.

The onset last year of hot flashes, albeit not severe, prompted a re-review of her situation. A mid-dose estradiol patch promptly relieved the flashes (Malinda was having more or less regular menses), but led to a noticeable increase in headaches. After a short hiatus, she again tried a much lower dose patch with fairly good hot flash relief. The poor quality sleep remained, however, and her physician recommended a Sleep Study.

Her polysomnogram showed an abnormal number (but not severe) of periodic limb movements, less REM sleep than normal, and some degree of sleep apnea. She has been scheduled for another study, this time with C-PAP. The idea is to compare the sleep study with and without C-PAP.

Malinda has no problem getting to sleep, or falling back asleep when she awakens, so sleep medications wouldn't be particularly helpful short-term. It is possible that long-term "hypnotic" therapy with diazepam (Valium®), lorezepam (Ativan®), etc. may help, but that's a road both she and I are loathe to embark upon.

Now that our son, Sam, sleeps through the night (even though he makes our bed his home most nights from 1-2 a.m. on) and with the distinct help from the patch and progesterone cream, Malinda's sleep quality is back to what it has been; she still requires a lot (but is more rested than she had been upon arising).

Perhaps the upcoming C-PAP study will offer a productive direction. Perhaps not. Malinda may be one of those individuals just past "the curve" who requires somewhat more than the average amount of sleep. I always knew she was "special."

*We have all passed a lot of water since then.*
—Samuel Goldwyn
(in discussion with Ezra Goodman)

# CHAPTER FIFTEEN

## YOUR PELVIC FLOOR...AND OTHER THINGS THAT FALL OUT

A newly available book[1] covers this topic in much better detail than I'll do here—but I'll try and give you a thorough overview. If urinary incontinence, pelvic organ prolapse, or interstitial cystitis is your issue, you definitely should buy this book.

### What Is Your "Pelvic Floor"? What Does it Do? How Can it Be Damaged?

Your "pelvic floor" is actually a muscular and fibrous diaphragm, held between bony structures (think trampoline) preventing things (like your bladder, uterus, vagina, rectum) from literally falling out. Through this diaphragm pass your urethra, exiting from the bladder; your vagina (with or without your cervix / uterus at its top) and your rectum, each held in place by their fibromuscular connections (see Figure 15-1).

"Pelvic relaxation," "prolapse," "cystocele," "rectocele"—there are several medical terms—is nothing more than one or more of these structures pushing, or herniating, through this diaphragm. Think of it as a hernia; nothing more, nothing less.

How can this fibromuscular "floor" be damaged; how can these herniations occur?

The biggest factor is our old friend, your genes. Some women have a tissue composition which simply predisposes them to pelvic relaxation.

It's more than that, of course. Although genetics alone is a factor in some instances of pelvic floor relaxation, other factors usually enter in as well.

Anything which tends to tear, separate, add excess pressure to or damage this diaphragm will, in a susceptible individual, predispose to pelvic relaxation. After genetics, these factors include:

---

[1] *The Incontinence Solution—Answers for Women of All Ages,* Wm. H. Parker, M.D., Amy E. Rosenman, M.D., and Rachel Parker; Simon and Schuster, 2002

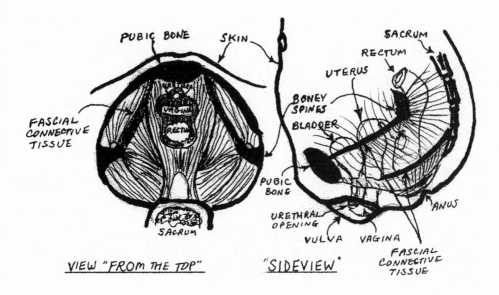

VIEW "FROM THE TOP"  "SIDEVIEW"

Figure 15-1. Cross-section and sideways view of pelvic organs and pelvic diaphragm. The area represented by thin lines are part of the muscular diaphragm.

1. <u>Weight</u>. The bigger you are, the more pressure there is on your pelvic diaphragm. Not much more to say...
2. <u>Smoking</u>. If you smoke, you probably cough. Chronically. Each cough puts a strain on the pelvic diaphragm. Cough, cough, cough. Do the math.
3. <u>Childbirth</u>. This is a hot topic, subject to much debate in the ob-gyn literature. If you've had a baby, you know the ripping, tearing, shearing pressure of passing an 8-lb. baby with a head the size of a cantaloupe through your poor unsuspecting vagina, through the pelvic floor. Bear down! Push! Puusshhh!!

In many areas (especially some South American and Middle Eastern countries), the primary (first time) c-section rate amongst the "upper class" population with access to prenatal care approaches or exceeds 75%. The major reason is to avoid pelvic floor damage.

Although the final verdict is not in, it makes sense that women who have not had the pelvic floor trauma of childbearing would be less likely, as they age and their tissue tone weakens, to have incontinence, prolapse, etc.

Again I must emphasize that although genetic factors are at work here, the more "traumatic" the birth (need for forceps, large episiotomy, etc.), the greater risk for later pelvic relaxation.

For this reason, an increasing number of women are considering requesting a primary cesarean section (before going into labor) to protect their pelvic floor. Obviously, childbirth does not automatically confer the curse of urinary incontinence and pelvic relaxation on the participant but, if the conditions are right (read: genetics; maybe add in excess weight and chronic cough, etc.) these conditions appear to be more likely in women who have had a baby/babies vaginally.

Extreme levels of exercise in the genetically-predisposed individual can also lead to pelvic relaxation, incontinence, etc.

## Why does incontinence and pelvic floor relaxation often manifest itself at midlife?

Urinary incontinence is a very common problem during and especially just after pregnancy and childbirth. The incidence, however, rises significantly around menopause and continues a slow rise thereafter. The reasons for this include:

1. Weight gain
2. Sudden decrease in estrogen levels. Estrogen helps maintain pelvic tissue tone
3. Aging tissue which finalizes the "payback" of childbearing.

## Consequences of Pelvic Floor Defects

1. Overall, the biggest problem is <u>urinary incontinence</u>, a condition in which a person leaks urine. Although there are several types of reasons for incontinence, "genuine stress incontinence" or "stress incontinence" (SI)—that is, involuntary loss of urine as a consequence of pelvic relaxation or "bladder droppage"—is the most common. (See below for other reasons for urinary incontinence.)

   In SI, an increase in intra-abdominal pressure caused by cough, laugh, exercise, etc. actually pushes the "bladder neck" (the lower part of the bladder) through your pelvic diaphragm, straightening it out and producing somewhat of a funnel for urine to leak through. It's usually worse or more likely to happen when your bladder is full. At the sign of a few drops of leakage, the person usually involuntarily tightens up their muscles, stopping the leak.

2. <u>Urinary retention</u>. Although much less common than urinary incontinence, if the bladder has really pushed through the diaphragm and is more or less continuously bulging out, it may be difficult to

empty properly without manual pressure through the vagina to push it back in. Urinary retention especially predisposes the individual to chronic infection in the turbid "lake" of the bladder. This leads to urgency.

3. <u>Prolapse</u>. Prolapse, or "symptomatic pelvic relaxation" is when one or more organs push through the diaphragm and, essentially, "hang out" (or almost so).

The more frequent offenders here are the uterus and bladder (frequently with one dragging down the other).

A "cystocele," also called a "cystourethrocele," is when the bladder (and frequently the urethra also) pushes through the diaphragm. If the rectum bulges through the posterior vaginal wall, the resulting prominent bulge through the lower part of the vagina is called a "rectocele." If your uterus has been removed and the vagina itself pushes down through the diaphragm, this is called an "enterocele."

Along with the bladder, the most usual organ to drop down is the uterus. The uterus is held in its place within the pelvis by poorly-formed "ligaments" (actually just a coalescence of connective tissue, not a true strong ligament) suspending the top of the uterus to the pelvic side wall ("round ligament") and the base of the uterus to the sacrum ("uterosacral ligament"). The "cardinal ligament" (just above the uterosacral) also helps secure the base of the uterus to firm connective tissue of the pelvic diaphragm.

If this tissue becomes less firm or these ligaments have been weakened or torn by childbirth or you are genetically challenged in the area of ligament strength, the uterus can prolapse, or slip through, the diaphragm into or through the vagina. Occasionally the whole thing can hang out.

4. <u>Anal Incontinence</u>. Anal incontinence is the uncontrolled passage of stool or gas, frequently without awareness. Although rare in younger women (although sometimes a consequence of tears during childbirth), 25-30% of women over 60 have some degree of anal incontinence!

Because it's so embarrassing, women rarely mention it to their doctors (which is unfortunate, because good treatments are available).

The usual cause of anal incontinence in women is injury to muscles or nerves of the pelvis and pelvic diaphragm during childbirth. The effects of aging on tissue tone (influenced by genetics) are also important.

## Causes of Urinary Incontinence Other than Pelvic Floor Defects
1. <u>Urge incontinence</u> ("irritable bladder," "dyssynergia").

"Urge" is caused by involuntary contractions of the muscles of the bladder, causing incontinence of small (but sometimes large) amounts of urine. This is the type of incontinence where you don't quite make it to the bathroom on time; when you "gotta go right now"; when you lose urine to the sound of running water or during lovemaking. It also is worse with a full bladder.

Causes of urge incontinence include bladder infection, bladder irritants (especially coffee, tea, acidic foods, etc.), and frequently the low estrogen levels that accompany menopause.

2.  Fistula. This is a rare cause of incontinence occurring after incomplete healing of a vaginal injury involving the bladder, or as a consequence of advanced bladder cancer.

    In this condition, occurring usually after a hysterectomy with inadvertent injury to the bladder (especially in a diabetic), the repair incompletely heals and an opening occurs between the vagina and the bladder resulting in constant urinary leakage ("wet all the time").

3.  Urethral diverticulum, also a rare cause in which an "out-pouching" or "diverticulum" occurs within the urethra, resulting in periodic discharge of very small amounts of urine from the diverticular "pocket."

4.  Neurological causes. If something (diabetes, major pelvic surgery, especially pelvic cancer surgery) injures or adversely affects the function of the nerve supply to the bladder, the bladder "doesn't know that it's full" and urine can be lost "off the top" via overflow.

## Workup of Urinary Incontinence

What should you expect your physician to do as a minimum, and under what circumstance should additional work be done? (Being "too busy" or being part of an HMO is no excuse for an inadequate workup.)

When should you have a workup? If involuntary loss of urine is embarrassing or interferes with your day-to-day activities, its cause should be investigated.

1.  A careful history and physical exam is the mainstay of urinary incontinence detective work. This includes questions and an exam in the doctor's office as well as any urological questionnaires that your health care practitioner may use.

    How long has this been going on? Under what circumstances do you lose urine? How much? What relationship does a full bladder have?

2.  Your doctor may ask you to fill out a "bladder diary" in which, more or less for 3 days, you list all your fluid intake, when and how much you void (including at night) and when, how much, and under what circumstances you leak urine. This can usually help her/him to figure out what is going on.

3. Your physician will need to differentiate between stress incontinence and urge incontinence, as well as to rule out other rare causes. (Remember, "stress incontinence" is caused by pelvic floor relaxation.) Frequently, both types of incontinence can occur together. If by your history and bladder diary it appears that stress incontinence is the problem, or part of the problem, this can be confirmed by basic office "urodynamics." In this testing, your doctor should have you empty your bladder, then catheterize you to see if you are retaining any urine. He or she may also culture the urine to rule out infection. He/she will then fill the bladder with water to see how much it holds, whether there are spasms, and also to demonstrate leakage when you cough, as well as confirm that "lifting up" the base of the bladder does indeed produce continence. A "q-tip test" may also be done, placing a q-tip in the urethra and checking its angle (to see if the bladder has "fallen") when you cough or strain.

4. When is other, more sophisticated (translation: electronics; bells and whistles) testing warranted? Some gynecologists, most urologists, and all urogynecologists do more sophisticated electronic urometrics and urodynamics, in which sophisticated instruments are utilized to more accurately tell what is really going on.

   Advanced urodynamic testing is not required the majority of the time. When is it a good idea?
   a. If you've had a previous incontinence operation that's failed
   b. If you're older than 70 (more or less)
   c. If there appears to be a "mixed" component to your incontinence and the urgency part is not easily controlled with medication
   d. Any time "things don't add up" in your workup; when the results of basic testing are confusing or contradictory.

5. <u>Cystoscopy</u>. Cystoscopy is looking inside the bladder with a tiny telescope. It is a quick and relatively painless procedure, usually done in the urogynecologist's or urologist's office. It is frequently a part of a thorough urodynamic workup, and is a good idea any time urgency or repeated infections are part of the equation.

6. <u>Ultrasound</u> may be utilized to check for complete (or incomplete) bladder emptying.

## Treatment of Incontinence

1. Nonsurgical approaches

   a. <u>Urgency</u>
   Here, lifestyle changes combined with medications are the mainstays of therapy.

What can you do (other than meds) for an "irritable bladder"?

Drink plenty of water. Carry a bottle in your car; one in your workplace; a cup by faucets at home.

It may seem paradoxical to drink lots of liquids when you have an incontinence problem, but dilute urine is less irritating to the bladder than when the urine is concentrated (but don't drink within 4 hours of bedtime or you'll be up all night!).

Certain foods can contribute to urinary urgency and frequency and discomfort. If bladder symptoms are related to dietary factors, strict adherence to a diet eliminating irritants should bring relief within 10-14 days. Once you are feeling better, you can begin to add foods back into your diet, one at time, to see if the problem returns. Remember to drink plenty of water as you add back foods.

These foods are acidic and considered irritants to the bladder:

| | |
|---|---|
| alcoholic beverages | guava |
| apples and apple juice | peaches |
| cantaloupe | pineapple |
| carbonated beverages | plums |
| chili and spicy foods | strawberries |
| citrus fruit | (sugar) |
| chocolate | tea |
| coffee (including decaf) | tomatoes |
| cranberries and cranberry juice | vitamin B complex |
| grapes | vinegar |

Bladder Retraining. Also known as "timed voiding." Here, you control your bladder rather than it controlling you. If you're tired of your bladder dictating when and where you must empty it, take over that control by timing your voids.

Start by going to the bathroom once every hour (get a wristwatch with an "hourly tone" if that helps). If that is successful, try going to every 2 hours. The idea here is to empty the bladder before its fullness causes reflex spasm (also, if stress incontinence is part of your problem, you'll find that you are much less likely to leak if your bladder is not full).

Timed voiding is helpful for both urgency and stress incontinence.

Medications. If these lifestyle changes do not offer considerable relief, meds can be a godsend. With some of the earlier medications, it was a little like trading a headache for an upset stomach, or in this case urgency for dizziness, constipation, some blurry vision and a dry mouth. Newer medications are now available which both last longer and offer fewer adverse effects.

Your health care practitioner can offer you several different medications, all of which function to "relax" the muscles of the bladder. These include oxybutanin (Ditropan®), now available in a sustained release form; toltaradine (Detrol®), and the "oldies but goodies" imipramine (Tofranil®) and hyoscyamine (Levsin®). Imipramine® is also good when taken at bedtime to ease nocturia (getting up lots of times at night to pee).

Although there are some medications used to treat overflow incontinence (from urinary retention), they are not all that good and frequently self-catheterization is necessary.

### b.　Stress incontinence

SI occurs when the muscles around the urethra and base of the bladder aren't strong enough to "keep the faucet closed," especially with cough, exercise, etc. A couple of decongestants such as pseudoephedrine (Sudafed®) or phenylpropanolamine (Ornade®, Dimetapp®) can occasionally be helpful for really bad days, but in general "drugs" do little to help SI.

The mainstay of nonsurgical therapy for SI is a combination of lifestyle changes and pelvic floor exercises, and both are worth a serious look, even if you are sure you're going to need surgery. Even if you're "going under the knife," they have beneficial effects in better preparing you and your tissues for the surgery.

Weight. The more you weigh, the greater is the downward pressure on your pelvic organs. The greater the pressure, the greater the likelihood they will "fall," prolapse, be incontinent, etc. and the greater that any repair of these problems will, in the long run, fail. Sorry...

Cigarette smoking leads to a chronic cough. The repeated pelvic pressure caused by a chronic cough does the same thing as excessive weight. (My God, how many reasons there are not to smoke!)

"Kegels" exercises. Good ol' Kegels. You all know what they are, but rarely do them. Kegels are a little like "diets": women do them for awhile, get some benefit, and quit.

What is a "Kegel"? What does it do?

The Kegel (named for for California gynecologist Dr. Arnold Kegel), or pelvic squeeze (love that term), is an isometric exercise of the levator muscles of the pelvic diaphragm, designed to build up and strengthen the pelvic floor. Although Kegels do little to help once incontinence is severe or "things have fallen out" (a little like closing the barn door after the cows have escaped), they can work well to control milder incontinence situations and, in any case, will strengthen the muscles to improve the outcome of later surgery, should it be necessary.

How do you do a Kegel? Imagine that you are waiting for the man who delivers a million dollars to come to your door. You wait. You have to pee.

You wait some more. You <u>really</u> have to pee. You hurry to the bathroom for a quickie and just after you start (Ahhhh!) <u>the doorbell rings</u>! What you do next to hurriedly stop the flow and rush to answer the door is a "Kegel."

If you're still uncertain, go to the bathroom, wash your hands and place two fingers well into your vagina. Tighten your vaginal and anal sphincter muscles (Squeeze!). You should feel a slight gripping on your fingers. You've just done a Kegel. If you try and try and... "no grip," see your health care practitioner or physical therapist for help.

How often should you Kegel? How long? How to remember? Here's a pearl: get 10 or so small pressure-sensitive labels (those peel-off white rectangles or dots). Write the word "Kegel" or "squeeze" on each. Put them everywhere: on the speedometer or display panel on your car. On the toilet paper holder and medicine cabinet mirror in your bathroom. On your makeup mirror and underwear drawer in your bedroom.  On the microwave and near food preparation areas in your kitchen. On the corner of your computer screen or picture of your husband and kids at home or at work. You get the picture.

Then, every time you see it, SQUEEZE as hard as you can for as long as you can. (You won't be able to hold it for more than 5-10 seconds. Do a bunch until you get bored. No one knows you're doing it. (Besides, the only other people who know what a Kegel is are other women who have been told by <u>their</u> doctor to squeeze.) Taking Kegels one step further, there are specially made weighted vaginal "cones" you can insert into your vagina and see if you can hold them in place with your Kegels. An experienced physical therapist can help you with this.

If your muscles just don't seem to want to do the squeezing, your health care practitioner or physical therapist can help. Biofeedback can also be helpful here.

Kegels also function in the area of bladder retraining. While the woman with SI usually coughs, leaks, and <u>then</u> squeezes, a "kegel-trained" individual may, when she knows a cough, laugh, or impact is imminent, <u>squeeze first</u>, cough—and not leak.

<u>Pessaries</u>. A pessary is a specially shaped silicon (usually) or rubber ring, sling, donut, cube, or inflatable ball, which is fitted into the vagina to, basically, hold things up. It doesn't cure things. It doesn't make it go away. (Out of sight, out of mind?) It can be an excellent temporary measure while awaiting surgery, or permanent measure if, for some reason or another, surgery is out of the question.

Pessaries come in many shapes and sizes. Not everyone can wear a pessary (you have to have a certain amount of vaginal muscle tone for it to be held in place). Ask your health care practitioner.

c.   <u>Overflow</u>

SI occurs when the muscles around the urethra and base of the bladder aren't strong enough to "keep the faucet closed," especially with cough,

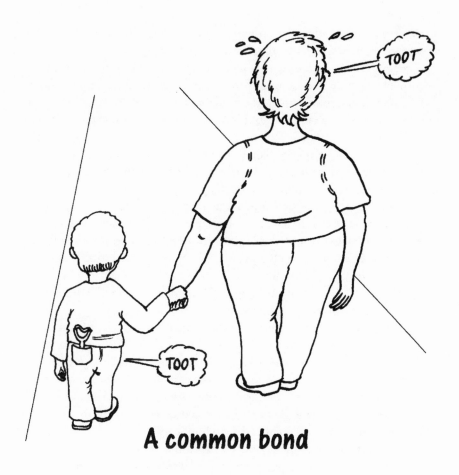

## A common bond

exercise, etc. A couple of decongestants such as pseudoephedrine (Sudafed®) or phenylpropanolamine (Ornade®, Dimetapp®) can occasionally be helpful for really bad days, but in general "drugs" do little to help SI.

2.  Surgical Approaches

Textbooks are written on this specific subject alone. In the interest of space, I shall not discuss surgery for stress incontinence in any great detail here.

Suffice it to say that although there are a great many different operations for the same problem, the choice of procedure and the care in which it is performed is of utmost importance for good long-term results (see "Choice of Surgeon" later in this chapter).

Operations for uterine prolapse. Hysterectomy, usually performed through the vagina is the procedure of choice for prolapse. In the circumstance of a woman who very much wishes to retain her uterus, a uterine suspension with added support from the lower uterine ligaments can be performed very well laparoscopically (tiny incision).

Operations for cystocele. (Bladder falling out.) An "anterior repair" is performed vaginally to decompress the bladder bulge, rebuild a new "floor" and frequently to repair tears in the fascial attachments. "Anterior repair" is a great operation for a cystocele, but is inadequate if incontinence is also part of the equation.

Operations for rectocele. Same practically as for cystocele, but in this case it is the vaginal floor and the "ceiling" over the rectum that is repaired. It can be performed vaginally or laparoscopically.

Operations for enterocele and vaginal prolapse (where the top of the vagina falls down) are varied. All involve supporting in some way (by suture or mesh ribbon) the top of the vagina to some tough ligamentous tissue, connected to an immovable object (bone). They can be performed vaginally, abdominally, or laparoscopically.

Operations for stress incontinence. How many they are! The best are divided into two categories: suspensions and slings.

The best suspension operation is the "Burch repair," performed either abdominally or laparoscopically, where sutures, mesh, or "anchors" are placed into the tough connective tissue around/under the vagina and urethra, on either side of the urethra, and connected to the tough connective tissue on the underside of the pubic bone. This is a lot like a swing and its chain. The chain is suspended from the pole above and anchored on each side to the seat. The seat is called the endopelvic fascia. By pulling it up (sutures) it supports the urethra and bladder base (the person sitting on the swing).

There are many types of slings and many different materials utilized. The newest, and from all appearances best, is utilizing a non-reactive synthetic mesh ribbon inserted through the vagina via a small incision on either side of the urethra, going up and passing just under the pubic bone and anchoring through the abdominal muscles and their connective tissues. This material is designed so it can pass up, but not slide down. Furthermore, after a short while, tissue ingrows into the spaces of the mesh, providing a further anchoring. TVT ("tension free vaginal tape") is one of these materials.

Although a "retropubic suspension" or TVT-type sling are the present "gold standards," that is not to say that other operations (and operations to come) don't have their place in certain situations.

An "anterior repair," repairing the base of the bladder only via a vaginal operation is inadequate surgery for stress incontinence (due to pelvic floor relaxation) in this day and age!

Collagen injections (transvaginally into the tissue around the urethra) is an extremely useful procedure in selected situations, especially when there is "funnelling" of the bladder outlet, repeated surgical failure, or when there are older or fibrotic tissues. The downside of collagen is that the injections must be repeated every couple of years.

## How to Pick the Right Doc for You

An official, board-certified urogynecologist (urogynecology is the latest officially recognized OB-GYN subspecialty) is usually an assurance of someone who knows what she/he is doing. But many other experienced practitioners (gyn or urologists) also know what they're doing and are excellent choices.

Questions to ask your practitioner:

(1) "What procedures do you use for stress incontinence?" Right answers include <u>Burch procedures</u> (open or laparoscopically), <u>TVT</u> or equivalent "sling" operation. A wrong answer is "anterior repair" (although this <u>is</u> a good operation for repairing a cystocele—bladder falling out— without incontinence.

(2) "What do you do for prolapse, cystocele and rectocele?" Right answers are vaginal hysterectomy with anterior and posterior repair, sometimes paravaginal repair and some method of support of the vaginal vault. Right also is a laparoscopic procedure to accomplish the same, if your gyn is an experienced laparoscopist (this can be assured if he/she is accredited by the Accreditation Council on Gynecologic Endoscopy).

(3) "What do you do for prolapse of the vagina?" Right answer is suspension by the sacrospinatus ligament (vaginally) or an abdominal or laparoscopic operation which suspends the top of the vagina by attaching it to the uterosacral ligaments (if strong enough), or by a mesh ribbon to the inner surface of the sacrum.

Ask questions! If your surgeon just schedules you for surgery without a workup and without full discussion with you, I'd <u>avoid that surgeon</u> and find someone more thorough who gives you an understandable, satisfactory explanation.

Let me emphasize: this chapter is the briefest of overviews and in no way fully covers the subject of pelvic relaxation and urinary incontinence. If incontinence especially is one of your issues, by all means get Dr. Parker's book, "The Incontinence Solution" and ... "read all about it"!

## MICHAELA'S STORY

"My bladder is between my legs," was Michaela's response when I asked her my standard, "What brings you here?"

Michaela looked a bit younger than her 71 years and she'd been to see several different physicians in the course of the last 3 years that she'd been increasingly bothered by this unwanted intrusion (or...extrusion). She had not found anyone who would explain things to her. Plus, she was scared to death of surgery.

Although she'd already seen several physicians, She still wanted an adequate "second opinion."

"I'm a very active person. I used to garden a lot and lift sacks of fertilizer but this thing has certainly put the damper on that. I used to be able to push it back in and it would stay, more or less, unless I strained or lifted. But now it's pretty much out. I push it in, but out it pops!"

She complained of bloating and low back pain (both common in cases of complete prolapse).

"If I don't push it in, I can't pee. I've tried three different pessaries. That balloon one did help, but I'm not sure I want to wear it all the time. I'm still limited in strenuous activities. And I pee sometimes when I cough or strain. I have to wear a pad, dammit! It seems I'm always pushing or stuffing or leaking. It embarrasses me."

Michaela was sexually active, I discovered during my workup. "Peter and I have been married only 5 years. We enjoy each other's company in more than one way. But this prolapse thing has definitely limited our love-making."

She was in good general health, she told me. She was taking Estrace®, Prometrium® and Synthroid® as well as numerous co-enzymes, vitamins, and "adrenal support supplements." She had had a uterine suspension 45 years previously, causing me to further suspect genetics at work here (Michaela weighed 118 lbs. and was a non-smoker. She didn't have many of the usual risk factors.)

On exam, she wasn't kidding: her bladder (with her uterus right behind it) was, truly, between her legs. It protruded, in all its pink glory, at least 2-3" outside the vagina.

Because of her age and the rather complicated nature of her situation (complete prolapse, some urinary retention, occasional incontinence and the previous surgical suspension), I suggested complete urodynamic testing and referred her to Chuck Armisty, a local urogynecologist whom I trusted.

After waiting 2 months (and my waiting an additional month to get reports) her testing was completed and included uroflometry, urethroprofilometry, voiding studies, urocystometry, and cystoscopy (the "whole 9 yards").

She was found to have a bladder infection (probably from the urinary retention as a consequence of her large, prolapsed bladder, which was treated with Cipro®. She was also found to have a degree of "detrussser instability" (urgency), probably caused by the chronic irritation caused by the prolapse and infection. Her urinary incontinence was worrisome both on the surface and because, after removal of her prolapsed uterus and decompression/repair of the cystocele, it was very possible that a fixation and "straightening" of the urethra would occur, worsening the incontinence. A suspension procedure (TVT or Burch) was recommended.

Additionally, in view of her severe prolapse and generally poor tissue tone, some sort of procedure to fix and suspend the apex of the vagina was recommended.

Although not significantly symptomatic, Michaela also had a modest rectocele (rectum bulging through the vagina), which would only get worse with time.

And she was sexually active. After fixing all of this, she needed to end up with a well-functioning vagina.

We discussed all of this in detail at a 45-minute follow-up visit. I gave Michaela the choice of either having me or Dr. Armisty do her surgery. Since the whole procedure could be approached through the vagina, there was no sense in doing a Burch suspension, which required an abdominal incision or laparoscopic approach, and I recommended the TVT. Since I have not been trained with TVT, I told her that if I were to do the rest of the surgery, I would call on the assistance of Dr. Pete Carroll, a local urologist who had over 100 TVTs under his belt.

Because of her age, I had Michaela see a cardiologist for a complete workup prior to her operation. She did have a couple of cardiac problems, but nothing significant, and she was cleared for surgery.

After her workup and the decision for surgery, Michaela was a nervous wreck and called me several times for reassurance.

Due to a combination of factors (Michaela felt comfortable with me, and Dr. Armisty didn't have time on his schedule for 2 months), Dr. Carroll and I did the surgery (a combination vaginal hysterectomy and enterocele repair, anterior and paravaginal repair, posterior repair, and sacrospinatous ligament vaginal suspension, as well as the TVT sling placement). In plain English, this is removing the uterus, closing off a "pouch" where the intestines can prolapse, pushing the bladder up, repairing the fascial connective tissue separation and "building up" a new connective tissue and muscular "floor" for the bladder, doing the same for the rectum (in this case, building a new "ceiling") and putting a strong permanent stitch into the ligament connecting the bony spines with the sacrum and anchoring it to the apex of the vagina for support, and also placing the TVT sling under the urethra. And (importantly) making sure there was still enough room for her Sweetie's member.

Michaela was in hospital for 3 days after her surgery. Her Foley catheter (bladder drainage tube) was removed on her second post-op day and she peed like a champ. She went home on her third post-operative day, hardly turning a hair. She was a bit anemic from blood loss at surgery and a small, self-contained leak in the area of surgery post-operatively, but this would correct itself with iron and vitamins.

Michaela is now 3 months out from her surgery. She has her spring garden in. Everything is staying in place. And after quite a bit of reticence (and 2 months ), she has proven the "functionality" of her vagina.

We both heaved a sigh of relief.

*I can't believe I forgot to have children..*
—Unknown

# CHAPTER SIXTEEN

## MIDLIFE AND CHILDLESS

Midlife is also a time when a not insignificant percentage of women face the fact that they do not have, and may not ever have, children (It is also a time that many midlife women with teenagers wish they were among the childless ranks.)

Frequently, this is accepted and reflects a decision made years previously, but many times the realization is a shock.

Waiting longer for babies may mean not having them at all. This may be OK and planned, or may be something which "just slipped on by" and is now perhaps beyond your grasp.

Many women temporarily put off childbearing for their careers, "climbing the corporate ladder." It's their 15-year plan: you work your tail off for a dozen years, get married somewhere along the line, have children in your late 30s or so. Sometimes that may slide into the early 40s. Many think that women regularly have babies into their 40s... no problem.

The fact is, fertility declines with age faster than modern pop culture has suggested. By age 42, almost 90% of a woman's eggs are chromosomally abnormal, most of them incapable of being fertilized (and when they are, with a higher rate of abnormal pregnancies). Certainly, the fertility percentage of a woman in her mid 30s is less than 50% of a woman at age 25. A woman's reproductive pinnacle is at age 27, with fertility falling off thereafter. By her late 30s, this percentage is 25%; by 42-43, it's down to less than 5% of her 20-something counterpart.

According to the last census, one in five United States women between the age of 40 and 44 are childless; of high-achieving women earning $100,000 or more a year, almost 50% have no children!

Despite miracle advances in so many areas of medicine, the inevitable biological clock ticks on. Seeing medical miracles in women in their 50s (even 60s) having babies, many women have come to think that there is no problem having babies in their 40s.

Yes, midlife women can have babies, but the options for women over 40 are often limited to using donor eggs or surrogates.

Also unfortunate is how these biological facts collide with competing messages faced by both men and women building careers.

Many women consciously pick a career over having children. But many women don't. "...the time just came and went... By the time it was too late, I didn't know it was too late..."

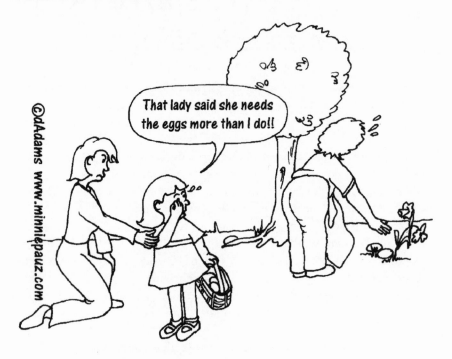

Additionally startling are pregnancy outcome statistics for women over the age of 40. The miscarriage rate climbs precipitously and is over 1 in 3 by the early/mid 40s. Likewise, the rates of preterm birth, pregnancy-induced hypertension (toxemia) and c-section also soar. The risk of having a child with trisomy-21 (Downs Syndrome) is 1 in 200 at age 37/38. This increases to 1 in 100 at age 40. By age 45 it's more than 1 in 25.

The odds of a genetic disorder increase steeply in women by their late 30s and early 40s—especially into their mid 40s.

As women age, so do their partners. The increased genetic mutational liability shouldered by midlife women extends to their male partners as well. Among other maladies, the rate of schizophrenia, for example, in adult offspring of "older" men increases precipitously, especially when these fathers are in their late 40s, 50s and 60s.

## Cryopreservation of Ovarian Tissue

Cryopreservation (freezing) of potentially fertilizable eggs could have great value for women undergoing egg-toxic chemo- or radiation therapy, or for those women who wish to forego childbearing until their 40s.

Although fertilized human embryos have been successfully frozen for many years (and successfully used in most in vitro fertilization {IVF} programs) the successful cryopreservation of human unfertilized eggs has been elusive; the reporting of successes has been relatively few and far between. This is surprising, since cryopreservation has been performed in other mammalian eggs for quite some time.

New work is being done presently with freezing actual ovarian tissue (collected usually by laparoscopic, tiny incision, biopsies) isolating primordial and primary follicles, and successfully cryopreserving these cells (although fertilizability and embryo normality is still unknown).

Look for this work to continue. I predict the time is not far off when women will be able to cryopreserve either individual eggs, or a small portion of ovarian tissue, for later fertilization and IVF embryo transfer.

So, to the 25-30% of you reading this book who are childless: you are not alone. Hopefully it is by choice. If by chance, and if you want it badly enough (and have the funds to see it through), consult your local gyn reproductive endocrinologist (fertility specialist). SART (The Society of Advanced Reproductive Technologies, http://www.sart.org, (205) 978-5000) can advise you where to find someone who can help.

The take-home message: choose, or biology will do it for you.

*I have lost friends, some by death...others through sheer inability to cross the street.*
—Virginia Wolf, *The Waves*

*Lord forgive all the little tricks I play on you and I'll forgive the great big one you played on me.*
—Robert Frost

*Everything is funny as long as it's happening to someone else.*
—Will Rogers

# CHAPTER SEVENTEEN

## BIG ODDS 'N ENDS

Chronic Fatigue and Fibromyalgia; Irritable Bowel Syndrome; Vulvodynia (Vulvar Pain Syndromes); Interstitial Cystitis; Depression

These quotes sum up, better than all my words to follow, the visceral feelings of women who, on a daily basis, have to deal with one or more of these maladies.

As in other topics discussed on these pages, a complete book can be written (and books have been) on each of these important areas.

I cannot hope to cover each completely. But what I can do is increase awareness and acknowledge that each of these entities is very real, does exist, and can be devastating for the one having to deal with them. Most importantly, for those of you suffering in silence from one or more of these problems, I hope this helps to give voice to your symptoms and point you in the right direction for help!

There is a very real thread connecting each of these maladies, which tend to begin prior to midlife, continue through the 40s, but luckily tend to fade as one ages past menopause.

Although perhaps less so with depression, the common bond here is a failure of the immune system to do its job in a specific area. What happens to rob one of energy as seen in chronic fatigue; to fail to clear toxins from the muscles in fibromyalgia? Why does the bladder wall of patients with interstitial cystitis (IC) fail to protect itself from the sting of its own urine?

What produces the inflamed nerve endings and faulty biofeedback in the different forms of vulvar pain syndromes?

In my experience, some significant emotional trauma appears to have been present in the lives of many of the women with the syndromes discussed in this chapter. Childhood or partnership abuse (emotional, physical or sexual) is frequent.

Why is a woman with one of these syndromes frequently afflicted by another? Why are these illnesses so often "bedfellows"?

I trace my theory back to the development (or lack thereof) and maintenance of immune function and what I strongly believe are adverse effects caused, simply, by how we were raised and the psychological and physical trauma that passage may have engendered.

There are those of us who are lucky to have been raised in a nurturing, caring environment, free from yelling, undue pressure, unreasonable demands, put-downs, and sexual, physical or psychological assault. There are those of us who weren't so lucky. And from this latter group come the recruits that this chapter speaks to.

Assuming this theory to be at least partially correct (as I obviously have), what can one do first to "stop the bleeding" and later to both understand the cause, the natural history of the situation, gain deeper understanding, hopefully getting nearer to the root of the problem.

You can't do anything about your genetics or your upbringing, but you can gain understanding and (better late than never), take charge of your destiny!

**FATIGUE AND PAIN YOU CAN'T EXPLAIN:** Chronic fatigue and fibromyalgia.

### Chronic Fatigue Syndrome.

Chronic Fatigue Syndrome (CFS) and fibromyalgia are different, but related, and may be corners of the same bed.

CFS is a state of significant longstanding fatigue in the face of otherwise appropriate good health and adequate sleep.

CFS is a diagnosis of exclusion, which means that there is no specific diagnostic test for the syndrome, although a number of CFS sufferers test positive for the Epstein-Barr virus (an easily available lab test). Although the diagnosis may be made in its absence, a positive test can be confirmatory.

Chronic Fatigue Syndrome is what its name implies: chronic tiredness without appreciable cause. No get up and go. Difficulty accomplishing daily chores (much less holding down a job). "All tired out" by only minimal activities.

As I said, CFS is a diagnosis of exclusion. If peri-menopausal symptoms seem to coincide with (or exacerbate) your fatigue, you must first adequately treat these symptoms and see what remains.

Many of the symptoms of CFS coincide with those of depression (and certainly the two can coexist; if I had Chronic Fatigue Syndrome, I'd probably be more than a little depressed!) Any fatigue workup should begin with an evaluation for depression. As a "screening tool," an instrument such as the Zung Self-Rating Depression Scale (SDS) (see Figure 17-1) is fine.

If it appears that a clinical depression is present, it should be treated by either your health care practitioner or a psychiatrist. If your fatigued state persists despite therapy, a true "fatigue workup" is in order.

The first order of business is to check your thyroid status. Typical symptoms of "low thyroid" include weight gain, fatigue, constipation, increased blood lipids and abnormal menses.

A TSH (or thyroid stimulating hormone test) is the most sensitive, although if you are on estrogen supplementation, a Free Thyroxin Index, or "FTI" should also be performed. In women with suspected autoimmune disease, your health care practitioner may also wish to test for anti-thyroid antibodies and/or thyroid microglobulins as part of your thyroid workup.

If the thyroid is OK, a complete workup for fatigue should include

1.  A CBC and ESR. CBC is a "complete blood count," or analysis of blood cells. The ESR test (also called the "SED rate,") is a very sensitive, but also very non-specific test of inflammation caused, perhaps, by altered immune function. If it is normal, you probably don't have altered immune function. If it's elevated, a thorough workup should follow.

2.  Liver function studies and hepatitis screens. Forms of hepatitis and other liver dysfunction can present as fatigue.

3.  Immune system tests such as lupus anticoagulant (LA), anti-nuclear antibody (ANA), Rheumatoid Factor (RF) and HIV testing (see also #1 above). Lupus especially can masquerade as chronic fatigue syndrome or fibromyalgia with symptoms of unexplained mood swings, energy loss, low grade fevers, facial flushing, etc.

4.  Tests for Lyme Disease.

5.  Stool cultures for candida (also known as the fungus monilia). Chronic systemic candidiasis can lead to fatigue-like symptoms.

6.  A "basic metabolic" or "chem panel" to quickly do an "all systems review."

If nothing turns up on the workup, or if items that are positive are treated and you are still fatigued, you probably have chronic fatigue syndrome.

So: how do you treat it?

# ZUNG SELF-RATING DEPRESSION SCALE (SDS)[5]

| Circle number in appropriate column. | A Little of the Time | Some of the Time | Good Part of the Time | Most of the Time |
|---|---|---|---|---|
| **1.** I feel down-hearted and blue | 1 | 2 | 3 | 4 |
| **2.** Morning is when I feel the best | 4 | 3 | 2 | 1 |
| **3.** I have crying spells or feel like it | 1 | 2 | 3 | 4 |
| **4.** I have trouble sleeping at night | 1 | 2 | 3 | 4 |
| **5.** I eat as much as I used to | 4 | 3 | 2 | 1 |
| **6.** I still enjoy sex | 4 | 3 | 2 | 1 |
| **7.** I notice that I am losing weight | 1 | 2 | 3 | 4 |
| **8.** I have trouble with constipation | 1 | 2 | 3 | 4 |
| **9.** My heart beats faster than usual | 1 | 2 | 3 | 4 |
| **10.** I get tired for no reason | 1 | 2 | 3 | 4 |
| **11.** My mind is as clear as it used to be | 4 | 3 | 2 | 1 |
| **12.** I find it easy to do the things I used to do | 4 | 3 | 2 | 1 |
| **13.** I am restless and can't keep still | 1 | 2 | 3 | 4 |
| **14.** I feel hopeful about the future | 4 | 3 | 2 | 1 |
| **15.** I am more irritable than usual | 1 | 2 | 3 | 4 |
| **16.** I find it easy to make decisions | 4 | 3 | 2 | 1 |
| **17.** I feel that I am useful and needed | 4 | 3 | 2 | 1 |
| **18.** My life is pretty full | 4 | 3 | 2 | 1 |
| **19.** I feel that others would be better off if I were dead | 1 | 2 | 3 | 4 |
| **20.** I still enjoy the things I used to do | 4 | 3 | 2 | 1 |
| Add up columns and tally for total raw score | | | | |

**Multiply raw score by 1.25 for SDS index score**

TOTAL RAW SCORE

x 1.25

SDS INDEX

Adapted from Zung.[5]

| SDS Index | Equivalent Clinical Global Impressions |
|---|---|
| Below 50 | Normal |
| 50-59 | Mild Depression |
| 60-69 | Moderate to Marked Depression |
| ≥70 | Severe Depression |

Adapted from Zung.[5]

= TOTAL RAW SCORE

Figure 17-1. Zung Self-Rating Depression Scale*
*Zung, W.N.K., "A Self-Rating Depression Scale." Archives of Clinical Psychiatry, 1965, Vol. 12, pgs 63-70.

There is no "magic bullet" for chronic fatigue syndrome (CFS). The mainstays of therapy are similar to those listed later in this chapter for fibromyalgia.

Believe it or not, exercise is probably the single best way to relieve symptoms. All three kinds of exercise-aerobic, muscle strengthening, and stretching-can help. (Using the "Goldilocks Principle": not too much, not too little, but just the right amount.)

Although moderation is important, working up to some degree of out-of-breath, sweaty exercise will work wonders.

The trick (and the difficulty) is to <u>start</u>. What's the last thing you feel like doing if you're fatigued? Exercise. Right.

Additionally, psychotherapy utilizing "cognitive behavioral therapy" can offer much needed support.

It's breaking a vicious cycle, really. You have to start somewhere. You <u>really will</u> feel better with 30-45 minutes of daily exercise. The difficulty is starting, promising yourself that you will drag your tired, achy butt to your machine or health club, etc. every day (or at least 4-5 times a week) for at least a 4-week trial. Give yourself a month.. See how you feel!

What about medication? Beyond therapy for other co-existing situations such as low thyroid, menopause, or other abnormalities, compounded preparations can be very helpful for CFS.

I am not going to give you a course in compounding here, but variable combinations including testosterone, DHEA, pregnenolone and possibly progesterone may be utilized. If general stress, "adreno-corticofatigue" (adrenal gland fatigue caused by long-standing states of stress) or autoimmune stress are part of your equation, pregnenolone administration either as a transdermal gel 25-50 mg/day or an oral capsule, 50-75 mg/day can help. Markers of adrenal fatigue can be a blood pregnenolone and/or salivary progesterone test. If both are low or in the low-normal range, pregnenolone may help.

Other medical help may include increasing your blood pressure if it is low, by increasing water and salt and utilizing medications known to increase blood pressure. A medication (Provigal®) utilized for narcolepsy can help a minority of CFS sufferers. An experimental drug specific for CFS now in phase III FDA trial, called Ampligen®, is showing promise. And many patients find a measure of relief in vitamins, herbs, and coenzymes.

A quite useful web site for CFS (as well as fibromyalgia) is http://www.drpodell.org.

## Fibromyalgia
Fatigue along with muscle soreness are common complaints. For women

who have fibromyalgia (as many as 7-8 million Americans), these problems become a way of life. For some it may be only a mild annoyance; for others it's a disability.

Although it has probably been around for centuries, fibromyalgia was recognized as an "official disease" only since 1990, when the American College of Rheumatology established criteria for doctors to use in making the diagnosis.

According to the American College of Rheumatology, what distinguishes fibromyalgia from other causes of chronic pain is the presence of "tender points"—specific distinct, sometimes swollen spots, especially on the back of the head, neck, upper chest, elbows, hips, knees, etc. that are painful when pressed. In all, 18 points have been identified; to fit the official criteria for fibromyalgia diagnosis, at least 11 points must be sensitive.

The original 1843 description of fibromyalgia as a "type of rheumatism with hard and tender places" still applies today. Make sure your doctor "maps" all of your tender points at your initial visit and follow-ups; this provides a visual and objective record to monitor changes at a glance.

Most fibromyalgia sufferers also experience a lowered pain threshold that makes normally tolerable levels of touch, heat and cold feel painful.

People with fibromyalgia may be sensitive to bright lights, loud sounds and stress, and subject to anxiety and fatigue; they also are more prone to headaches, irritable bowel syndrome, and interstitial cystitis (a severe form of irritable bladder—see later in this chapter...)

What causes fibromyalgia? No one knows exactly, although an alteration in immune function enters in here somewhere. It can develop gradually, or suddenly, weeks after a sometimes minor auto accident or injury. The common pattern of fibromyalgia is one of ups and downs, never disappearing entirely.

Some medication can help; several drugs have been shown to ease symptoms, but only work ⅓-½ of the time. A group of antidepressant medications called tricyclics, and especially amitriptyline (Elavil®) and nortriptylene (Pamelor®), but used in dosages of only 10-20% of the amount needed in depression, have the best track record and are a first line therapy, usually helping within days. Another group of antidepressants, the SSRIs (e.g., Prozac®, Paxil®) are less effective than tricyclics, but may be combined with them for relief.

Other medications which may give relief when the old standbys fail are gabapentin (Neurontin®), originally developed as an anti-seizure medication; the muscle relaxer tizanidine (Zanaflex®), and odansetron (Zofran®), used effectively to treat nausea and found to be useful for fibromyalgia in European studies.

Another theory on the therapy of fibromyalgia has been developed by R. Paul St. Armand, MD (www.guaidoc.com; www.guaifenesin.com). Dr. St. Armand theorizes that fibromyalgia is inherited and that trauma, infection or stress can aggravate it, but are rarely its cause. Almost 40 years ago, Dr. St. Armand found that the uricosuric medications used to treat gout (which cause urinary excretion of excess uric acid) helped patients with the ill-defined, multi-faceted illness which later became known as "fibromyalgia," and two gout medications (Probenecid and sulfinpyrazone) proved effective but had side effects.

A few years ago, Dr. St. Armand and his colleagues realized that the expectorant guaifenesin, which promotes the discharge of phlegm, was weakly uricosuric and, while not potent enough to treat gout, appeared to work extremely well for fibromyalgia.

Starting out at 300 mg twice daily was sufficient for approximately 20% of patients; at 600 mg twice daily another 50% appeared to improve and, at 1800 mg per day another 20% showed reduction of tender areas. Rarely, 2400 mg per day was necessary to adequately treat symptoms. In his studies, guaifenesin was distinctly more effective than previous medications and had no listed side effects. There is no patent on guaifenesin and it is inexpensive.

If trying guaifenesin, it is important to eliminate salicylates (compounds with aspirin) from your body, as guaifenesin is blocked by these compounds which may be ubiquitous in medications, cosmetics, shaving aids and oral hygiene products. These include aspirin and anything which has salicytic acid, salicylate or salicylamide in its ingredients, including many creams, balms, and lotions for muscle pain. Additionally, mint and mint oils, menthol, PeptoBismol and many plant derivatives contain salicytic acid derivatives. (See the web sites listed above for details).

Medication is only part of the story. How you live (lifestyle changes!) can mean the difference between only mild discomfort and disability.

As discussed under Chronic Fatigue, exercise is probably the single best way to relieve symptoms.

Also, do what you can to control stress. Stress aggravates fibromyalgia symptoms. Meditation, deep breathing, progressive muscle relaxation (see Chapter 13) can help alleviate stress.

Fibromyalgia sufferers should do their best to change thinking patterns that elevate stress. Worry and panic about small setbacks or feeling compelled to make up for bad days by overdoing it when one feels better are counterproductive. Sometimes just being aware of these pitfalls is a step toward avoiding them.

Important as well is keeping regular hours and getting adequate sleep. (See Chapter 14.) Massage and body work (including Rolfing and "myofascial release") can ease symptoms, but be careful to find a therapist who is experienced in treating fibromyalgia patients.

## IRRITABLE BOWEL SYNDROME

Irritable bowel syndrome, or "IBS" (called "spastic colon" in the past) affects an estimated 10-15% of Americans and is characterized by irregular bowel movements and recurrent wrenching, spasmodic abdominal pain and bloating, usually relieved by bowel movements. Although it can't be traced to a single organic cause and isn't life-threatening, the syndrome can wreak havoc in the lives of those who suffer from it.

Three groups can be identified: chronic, recurrent abdominal pain with constipation; with diarrhea; or with alternating constipation and diarrhea. Women are more affected than men (3-20 times); occasionally worsening of symptoms is noted when the progesterone is elevated (as in the latter part of the menstrual cycle or with high dose progesterone therapy).

Like other maladies described in this chapter, IBS is not fun to have!

IBS should be differentiated from colitis, Crohn's disease and diverticulosis/itis which, although they can coexist with IBS, are separate medical problems.

Officially, IBS has, as they say medically, "no identifiable cause." Doctors refer to it as a "functional" disease, but I think that's just a cop-out. IBS is definitely not in your head.

With IBS, as other like problems, certainly emotions and behaviors can make the disease better or worse (every emotion triggers biochemical changes in the body). With its predilection for stressed or Type A" individuals and its interrelationship with other disorders such as fatigue, interstitial cystitis, vulvodynia (discomfort around the vaginal opening) and depression, there must be an immune system thread in there somewhere.

Also, noting its prevalence in family members and generations, some sort of genetic and/or environmental/developmental relationship is probable.

Very interesting is the finding, in IBS sufferers, of a very large percentage who have suffered abusive relationships, especially childhood sexual abuse.

Stress is definitely related. Part of this is a "chicken and egg" thing (if you're stressed you're more likely to get IBS; if you have IBS, you're more likely to get stressed.), but life stresses and a stressful existence definitely seems to be among the causative factors (see Chapter 13).

Therapeutic measures can be divided into behavioral and medical. As in so many other areas of women's health, lifestyle changes are of paramount importance.

"To Heal the Body, First Prepare the Mind"

Stress reduction (Chapter 13) is important; most IBS sufferers will note exacerbations of their symptoms when they are stressed.

Also key are basic exercise and dietary changes, which go a long way towards quelling symptoms. These are:

1. Increase daily exercise
2. Increase daily intake of fluids, especially water
3. Significantly increase daily fiber: whole grains, fruit, legumes, etc. Fiber is "nature's broom" waiting to sweep you out from the inside. Fiber increases stool weight and speeds it through the intestine, as well as diminishing abdominal pain and stool frequency.
4. Decrease fatty foods, fried foods; keep red meats to a minimum.
5. One round tsp. of psyllium (the active ingredient in Metamucil) dissolved in a glass of water, juice, milk, etc. once-twice per day. Psyllium is cheap and, if drunk promptly after mixing with liquid, is entirely tasteless (but don't let it sit or it will become jelly-like). Available at any health food store.
6. If the psyllium doesn't quite do it, try Bulk Bran (also available at health food stores), 1-3 Tbs. daily, either over cereal or in a glass of water.

The use of enteric-coated peppermint oil capsules (available through certain health care practitioners, at some health food stores, or by calling Phytopharmica at 800-553-2370 and asking for "Mentheral") helps many with resistant IBS. Take 2 capsules 3 times a day between meals. Make sure they are "enteric-coated" or they'll cause heartburn.

The above measures will go a long way toward alleviating IBS symptoms. However, if they don't, several medications and other complementary and alternative medications are available, depending on symptoms: cramps; diarrhea; constipation. Additionally, some psychoactive drugs have found to be of benefit.

If cramps and painful spasms (with or without diarrhea or constipation) are still an issue after dietary changes and peppermint oil capsules have been tired, antispasmodics such as dicyclomine (Bentyl®) or hyoscymine (Donnatal®; Levsin®) may help. Only two drugs (both of which, incidentally, interact with seratonin receptors) are approved for treatment of IBS in women who don't respond to conventional therapy.

Tegoserod (Zelnorm®), FDA approved in 2002, is indicated for IBS sufferers with diarrhea. Alosetron (Lotronex®) is indicated for patients with constipation. Although briefly removed from the market, Lotronex returned in 2002 with revised prescribing guidelines.

If diarrhea is an issue, try loperamide (Imodium-AD®); if it's constipation try MOM or Miralax®.

Amitriptyline (Elavil®) 20-50 mg at hs; Desipramine (Norpramine®) in the same doses and more recently paroxitine (Paxil®), 10-40 mg per day are helpful to "quiet things down" if stress remains an issue.

Many herbs have been utilized with mixed success for IBS, including bistort (also called snakeweed and adderwort), fennel, flax, gentian, marshmallow, meadow sweet, and turmeric.

Please refer to any good herbal (see Chapter 20) for details.

## VULVODYNIA

"It burns." "It stings." "It feels like ground glass inside me." "I can't have sex (or if I do, I pay for it for hours and days afterwards)." "It just hurts."

Vulvodynia is a catch-all term which means, literally, vulvar pain (an aptly descriptive term). It has many facets and is actually several different disorders with one common thread; they all involve the vulva, all the symptoms wax and wane, are frequently not diagnosed or misdiagnosed, and likely have an immune system relationship.

Many doctors are still not familiar with vulvodynia and as a result many patients are misdiagnosed or go undiagnosed altogether. Since the pain of vulvodynia isn't always accompanied by visible skin changes, patients are sometimes told "it's all in your head." But the condition is very real!

The International Society for the Study of Vulvar Diseases (ISSVD) defines vulvodynia as chronic vulvar discomfort and pain, especially that are characterized by complaints of burning, stinging, irritation or a rawness around the vulva/vagina/rectum. Although burning sensations are the most common, the pain is highly individualized. It may be constant or intermittent, localized or diffuse. As with other chronic pain situations, it has a major impact on quality of life and frequently significantly affects one's ability to engage in sexual activity and can even interfere with daily functioning.

These limitations can affect self-image and sometimes lead to depression.

There are four basic types of vulvodynia and they are not always easy to distinguish from each other: Dysesthetic Vulvodynia, Vulvar Vestibulitis, Cyclic Vulvovaginitis (yeast related), and Vulvar Dermatoses.

1. <u>Dysesthetic Vulvodynia</u> is pain caused by irritated or inflamed nerve endings in the vagina and inner labia and may extend to the anus and groin area. Some women may experience sharp pains or deep aching. Dysesthetic Vulvodynia is more common in peri- and post-menopausal women and may also be seen in women with fibromyalgia and/or interstitial cystitis.

2. <u>Vulvar vestibulitis</u> is inflammation around the "vestibule" or opening to the vagina, and may occur alone or with other types of vulvar pain. Symptoms include sensations of burning and dry, raw, or tight skin.

Pain is usually caused by external touch, from pressure during intercourse, tampon insertion, tight pants, bicycling or horseback riding, etc.

The symptoms are variable, with some patients only having discomfort with intercourse, while others have pain on a daily basis, finding it difficult to sit or walk. Pain around the clitoris ("Clitoriynea") is not rare.

If the pain is severe and enduring, some women may develop vaginismus, a spasm of the pelvic floor muscles so severe that it makes intercourse or tampon insertion impossible.

Vulvar Vestibulitis patients tend to be younger, in their 20s and 30s. Vulvar Vestibulitis probably makes up the largest number of vulvodynia patients.

3. Cyclic Vulvovaginitis. Caused by the yeast, *candida*, it may affect the vulva without causing any obvious vaginal discharge, but causing pain, swelling, and occasional tearing. Symptoms may flare around the time of menses. Chronic yeast has also been proposed as one of the causes of Dysesthetic Vulvodynia.

4. Vulvar Dermatoses. Skin disorders which occur in this area may cause chronic itching or burning and, when scratched, these areas become inflamed, irritated and hypersensitive. They include *lichen simplex, lichen sclerosis, hypertrophic dystrophy* (with patches of toughened skin), etc.

What Causes Vulvodynia?

"The cause of vulvodynia is unknown." (Another one!) Usually when you hear this statement, you know that immune and psychological factors are at work. Speculation, however, revolves around:

- An injury to or irritation of the nerves of the vulva
- A hypersensitivity to *candida*
- An allergic response to environmental irritants
- An increased concentration of oxalic crystals in the urine
- Irritation or spasms of the muscles that support the pelvic organs.

There is no evidence the vulvodynia is caused by infection or is a sexually transmitted disease.

How is it diagnosed? Your history alone should suggest vulvodynia to an experienced practitioner (see later for help in locating one). In dysesthetic vulvodynia, the diagnosis is suggested by history and there may or may not be visible skin irritation and generalized sensations of itching and burning not related to touch or pressure.

The hallmark of vulvar vestibulitis is an exquisite sensitivity of the tiny gland openings at the entrance to the vagina (the "vulvar vestibule") when touched even with something as gentle as a q-tip (the so-called "touch test").

Many patients also have tiny red spots at the openings of the tender areas, the openings of the glands of the vulvar vestibule.

Even when *candida* is suspected of causing chronic vulvar irritation, it frequently is not picked up on vaginal cultures. It is thought that some women may develop hypersensitivity to even very low concentrations of *candida,* and "reinfect" themselves via the GI tract.

*Vulvar dermatoses* are skin disorders that cause either very thin, sensitive skin, occasionally with white patches (white vulvar dystrophy or lichen sclerosis) or hypertrophic, thickened reddened skin (hypertrophic or red vulvar dystrophy), possibly caused by the chronic irritation. A biopsy is frequently helpful in order to classify the lesion and choose proper therapy (as well as rule out malignancy in certain situations). It is also important to note that many vulvar irritations are caused by skin irritants (e.g., soaps, perfumes), allergic drug reactions, overuse of medications (especially topical steroids) or infectious causes such as herpes and HPV.

Who gets vulvodynia? Why? The $64,000 question. The demographics shake down as follows:[1]

Almost 70% of patients report a past history of yeast infection and almost all patients report other health problems including pelvic pain and bladder or bowel dysfunction.

The most common physical activity limited by vulvar pain is (obviously) sexual intercourse, although clothing choices, sitting and walking are also difficult for some vulvodynia sufferers. A majority of women often or always avoid sexual intimacy; after all, sex is supposed to be pleasurable!

Interestingly, a large percentage of patients have a post-secondary education and at least half have not given birth.

The average duration of symptoms prior to diagnosis was 32 months in this study!

There appears to be no increased incidence of sexual abuse or sexual assault among women with vulvar vestibulitis. It is noted that women with vulvodynia report increased gastrointestinal symptoms, headaches, and various other problems.

Since vulvodynia and especially vulvar vestibulitis is associated with a significant change in intimate lifestyle such as sexuality, intimate relationships and psychological well being, make sure you are comfortable with your practitioner and that (s)he is comfortable in relating to this important aspect of your condition.

---

[1]"The Demographic Profiles of Vulvodynia Patients," L.A. Sadowaik, M.D., National Vulvodynia Association News, Winter 1999

Some vulvodynia experts see an association of vulvodynia, especially vulvar vestibulitis, with the HPV virus, and a check or an HPV DNA test is a good idea when you have vulvar vestibulitis. This may be why some anti-viral agents like interferon (see below under "treatments") may be helpful in some women with recalcitrant vestibulitis.

Most patients experience a huge sense of relief once a concrete diagnosis is made, feeling reassured that their pain is real and that the condition is neither malignant or communicable.

Treating Vulvodynia

Although currently there is no cure for vulvodynia, treatments aimed at symptom relief include oral drug therapies such as low doses of tricyclic antidepressants, antihistamines or sedatives, anticonvulsants, local estrogen therapy, nerve blocks, interferon, biofeedback, dietary modifications and occasionally surgery. Another and frequently effective therapeutic approach is aimed at eliminating traces of candida from the body.

Specific conditions such as vulvar dermatoses (vulvar dystrophies) are more amenable to treatment. Therapy includes warm baths, soothing lotions, a nighttime sedative such as Atarax® to prevent itching, wearing cotton gloves at night to limit skin peeling from itching, and, of course, the mainstay of therapy, relatively potent steroid creams such as triamcinolone or TAC (first option) or clobetasol (Temovate®) if TAC doesn't work, or for more serious conditions.

Non-specific conditions such as vulvar vestibulitis and dysesthetic vulvodynia are more challenging; improvement may take weeks to months, and conditions wax and wane. What is initially helpful may become less so with time. Therapies may come and go, only to be helpful again. Spontaneous remission of symptoms occurs in some women, while in others multiple attempts at medical management fail to relieve all symptoms. No single treatment program is successful in all women; patients frequently become frustrated with the failure of their health care practitioner to identify a specific cause for their symptoms.

Both dysesthetic vulvodynia and vulvar vestibulitis are commonly and usually somewhat successfully treated with low doses (10-25 mg) of a tricyclic antidepressant medication known as amitriptyline (Elavil®) or nortriptylene (Norpramine®), although sometimes far larger doses are necessary. Gabepentin (Neurontin®), beginning at 100-200 mg at bedtime and going up from there frequently provides additional relief.

Another dietary approach which helps some sufferers is to minimize acidic foods (see list in Chapter 15). Dr. John Willems, a vulvar disease expert at Scripps in La Jolla, CA and others, feel that occasionally there may be an allergic environmental etiology which can perhaps be mitigated by the use of the drug hydroxyine in low (10 mg) doses.

Local vulvar hygiene is essential: keep the vulva dry, avoid vulvar irritants, rinse the vulva with plain, cool water after voiding, use mild soaps such as Neutragena® or Basis® while bathing, wear loose clothing (especially during exercise), rinse clothing thoroughly to remove detergent irritants, use only 100% natural (unbleached) cotton menstrual pads.

Topical estrogen cream is frequently helpful for vulvodynia and should be included in all initial regimens.

I've had good success with treating ("on spec") most all of my vulvodynia patients (especially those with vulvar vestibulitis) with a potent moniliacide. This usually involves two courses of double strength Terazol® cream, plus two weeks of daily fluconazole (Diflucan®) at 100 mg per day followed by 2 months of twice weekly 150 mg dosing.

Since chronic muscle spasm or tension is an automatic response to long-continued intense genital pain, biofeedback monitoring can help correct the spasms of the pelvic floor musculature, frequently relieving vaginal muscle spasms.

Oxalate crystals, which are normal byproducts of the body's metabolism and are excreted in the urine, are very acidic and can irritate the mucus membranes of the vulva when overproduced. For this reason, a diet low in high-oxalate foods, plus taking oral calcium citrate (which tends to neutralize oxalate crystals) twice daily or whenever high oxalate foods are consumed, may be helpful. High oxalate foods include all beans, beer, beets, berries, celery, chocolate, chard, eggplant, some grapes, green peppers, peanuts, spinach, squash and tofu, to name a few. There are ways to test for oxalates in the urine, but many patients simply try to lower the amounts of these foods and/or self-administer calcium citrate to see how it works.

Local vestibular injection of the anti-viral agent Interferon® (0.05 cc injected just under the skin of each lower labia majora twice weekly for 8 weeks) is sometimes effective when the general measures described above fail. It's definitely worth a try. It works best in patients who also test positive for the human papilloma virus (HPV).

Occasionally, local injection of steroids with a local anesthetic may help.

If all else fails to work, excellent successes have been achieved in vulvar vestibulitis with local excision (via a laser or otherwise) of the sensitive glandular area of the vulvar vestibule. Although this surgical procedure is frequently successful, it makes sense to try other less invasive methods first.

Most important, though, is treatment of the sexual difficulties encountered in practically all sexually active women with these conditions. This is not done in a vacuum and your partner should be brought into the mix.

If it hurts to even be touched, much less to make love, first something must be done to break the pain cycle (see all that's written above). When you are ready to participate again in sexual intimacy, two things are key: lubrication and analgesia.

You will get nowhere fast if you're dry, and saliva (although frequently fun getting there) is not the best lubricant in this situation. I'd try baby oil or one of the water-based lubricants such as Astroglide®. Copiously.

If it's still too uncomfortable, however, try a local anesthetic like Emla® cream or 5% topical lidocaine gel (both prescription items) 10-15 minutes before lovemaking. It helps numb the painful area without diminishing sexual pleasure. Also try applying to the area at bedtime/overnight.

Getting Information about Vulvodynia and finding a good health care practitioner

Two must-see addresses for women suffering from vulvodynia are:

1.  National Vulvodynia Association
    P.O. Box 4491
    Silver Spring, MD 20914
    Phone: 301-299-0775
    Web site: http://www.nva.org

2.  The Vulvar Pain Foundation
    P.O. Drawer 177
    Graham, NC 27253
    Phone: 336-226-0704
    Web site: http://www.vulvarpainfoundation.org

Check these web sites for the name of a good clinician near you. If you're having trouble finding someone who has the time and is up to date in diagnosis and treatment of vulvar pain syndromes, it's worthwhile to even travel some distance for care.

## INTERSTITIAL CYSTITIS

IC is a chronic inflammation of the bladder that strikes mostly younger and mid-age women (luckily it seems to dissipate after midlife). It leaves the bladder's lining bleeding, scarred, and unable to hold normal amounts of urine, causing severe and often unrelenting pain and the need to race to the bathroom as often as every 15 minutes night and day. Needless to say, work and travel are difficult for an IC sufferer. Indeed, the Social Security Administration has ruled IC incapacitating enough to legally render someone disabled!

There is no specific test for IC; diagnosis is made because of the symptoms and by ruling out everything else from infection to cancer. The patient may be put under general anesthesia to stretch the bladder wall in search for some of the classical signs.

If you suffer from severe urinary frequency and pain, have been treated with numerous courses of antibiotics and are no better, consider IC. Check the Interstitial Cystitis Association's web site (http://www.ichelp.com) or telephone (800-HELP-ICA) for information and a list of specialists who can help.

IC is greatly underdiagnosed and misdiagnosed as recurrent urinary tract infection, endometriosis, vulvodynia, adhesions, pelvic pain, etc. Pressing on the bladder produces tenderness as severe as the symptoms.

Probably about 22-3% or more of American women have some form of IC. If you have a problem with painful intercourse, premenstrual pelvic pain or vaginal pain along with frequent and/or urgent urination, IC should be on the top of your list. Potassium rich foods such as chocolate, coffee, citrus fruits and tomatoes are associated with symptoms flares.

Like vulvar pain syndromes, chronic fatigue and fibromyalgia, IC is chronic. Sufferers have good days and bad days.

What's most likely to help? Selecting a therapy for IC is a challenge. A medication that helps one woman may not help the next; some therapies work for awhile and then are ineffective, and then, surprisingly, are effective again...

The standbys: amitriptyline (Elavil®) in small doses given at bedtime and occasionally in the morning helps, as does Vistaril® (hydroxyzine) in a 50 mg dose, acting as a tranquilizer and "body relaxant" during the daytime. Frequently, pain medications such as codeine, Vicodin® or Percocet® are necessary. "Anticholinergics" (GI tract anti-spasmodics) such as Donnatol® and the Levsin® drugs frequently lead to relief for awhile.

Anti-spasmodics (Detrol®; Ditropan®) work in some, but usually do not provide significant help. Pentosan polysufate (Elmiron®) is the only FDA-approved oral therapy aimed at IC and improves symptoms by approximately 25-40%, but its full benefit may not be seen for 6-8 months.

Some alternative practitioners have found success utilizing marshmallow root tea, which contains starch, mucilage, pectin and calcium oxylate, among other components. Acupressure may help to relieve pain. DMSO, also FDA approved, is a fluid inserted into the bladder when oral agents fail. Given weekly for 6-8 week, it is effective for 40-60% of patients.

New on the horizon may be a test for a toxin called APF, or Antiproliferative Factors, which are churned out by bladder cells of IC patients. APF appears to decrease levels of a growth factor called HB-EGF that's important in producing cells necessary to repair damaged bladder lining, essentially producing a vicious cycle where the bladder harms itself and then blocks its own healing mechanism.

Hopefully, aids in diagnosis will be followed by more predictable therapies. However, many of the above-mentioned medications in combination or in sequence, provide considerable relief.

Lifestyle-wise, anything which serves to reduce stress (see earlier chapter) will also help with IC. IC is stressful. Stress weakens the immune system, which worsens IC. Worsening IC causes stress.

There are several ways you can block this cycle: (1) stress reduction work, meditation, healing visualizations, prayer; (2) be under the care of a health care practitioner who "gives a damn" about IC; (3) be in touch with the IC Association for support, information and other invaluable aids.

## DEPRESSION

The subject of depression weaves in and out of this book, as it frequently does through midlife for both men and women. Its presence, its relationships and its medications aren't new to you if you've gotten this far in "The Bible." With all of the changes and challenges that midlife has to offer, depression can be an occasional or a frequent companion.

The presence of this small corner of "The Bible" is to simply remind you of the presence and frequency of mood changes during midlife.

You should not be inattentive to how you feel. A mild depression is as potentially dangerous to you as any other illness is during its beginning stage.

Awareness. Knowing where to go and knowing available treatments so that you will be informed when you enter into a discussion with your health care practitioner to decide if therapy is indicated, if medication is indicated, and what are the options.

What are the options?

Several complementary and alternative medications and botanicals have been utilized both by native cultures and in the present day for treatment of depression. These include clary sage; gamma butyrolactone; ginseng; hops; khat; mistletoe; mugwort; SAM-e; St. John's wort and yerba maté. Among these, St. John's wort and perhaps SAM-e have proven the most effective.

An avalanche of peer-review, behavioral and clinical evidence speaks to the beneficial effects estrogens, more specifically estradiol, have especially on the mood/depressive symptoms seen in midlife.

Although the use of hormones is to some degree guided by clinical lore, studies both large and small have shown its benefit, at least short-term, for peri-menopausal depressive disorders.

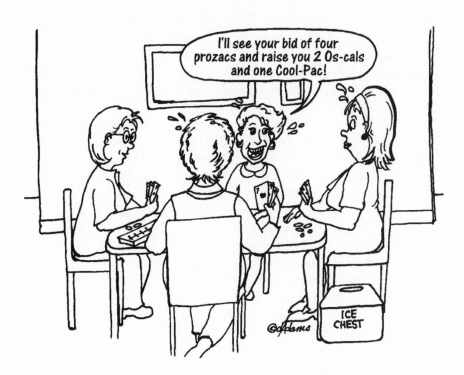

Although most estrogens are effective, many studies point especially to transdermal estrogen as perhaps the most effective and best tolerated mode of administration.

The use of estrogens for adverse mood symptoms beyond the transition into menopause is controversial. However, if, each time you attempt to wean off estrogen supplementation you find yourself depressed, you should discuss with your health care practitioner the pros and cons of staying on estrogen vs. taking up an anti-depressant while tapering off the estrogen. Also, the addition of estradiol to an SSRI appears in many women to be more effective than either one alone.

There is little literature outside of clinical reports that speaks to the role of bioidentical progesterone, either via oral micronized capsules, or cream/lotion. As it has no real downside, it certainly should be an option if your depression is resistant to other forms of therapy.

Hormonal treatment, once reserved only for hot flashes, peri-menopausal mood disorders and vaginal problems is now slowly finding a broader audience; some prophesy that within 20 years millions of women will be turning to it for psychological help.

Estrogens have been found, in many women, to be a stimulant, and vegetative depressions can sometimes be turned around by adding estrogen to the system.

Progesterone slows you down and, in proper doses, can be helpful for an agitated depression, or cyclic depressive symptoms when your progesterone level is low.

With regard to medication there are several "classes" of antidepressants. Some are old and some new. Each has its advantages and disadvantages. Following are the most utilized medications grouped together as types. This list is not complete.

Tricyclics. Tricyclic antidepressants include amitriptyline (Elavil®), desipramine (Norpramine®), imipramine (Tofranil®) and nortriptylene (Pamelor®). The advantages of tricyclics include low cost, long experience, and good results. Disadvantages are drowsiness and sedation in some, lowering of the blood pressure, occasional cardiac arrhythmia, diminution in sexual desire, weight gain and dry mouth.

SSRIs. Like the tricyclics, the group of SSRIs is made up of several medications, each with some advantages and disadvantages. Fluoxetine (Prozac®), paroxetine (Paxil®), sertraline (Zoloft®), citalopram (Celexa®), and fluvoxamine (Luvox®) are examples of "selective serotonin reuptake inhibitors," or serotonin enhancers, which act to prevent seratonin ("you remember…!"), a mood-elevating blood protein, from leaving the brain. SSRIs provide a relatively inexpensive means to treat depression in an outpatient setting. SSRIs are very effective in decreasing or eliminating depressive symptoms without sedation and don't cause dry mouth, blood pressure abnormalities, cardiac difficulties or excessive weight gain. Disadvantages include nausea (which usually disappears in 2-3 weeks, especially if your medication is taken with food), sexual dysfunction (diminished desire and difficulty achieving orgasm), and insomnia (in ±15% of patients). This insomnia can usually be mitigated by decreasing the dose or adding in a low dose of Trazodone® (another antidepressant and sedative taken at bedtime).

The SSRIs are similar to each other, but Paxil® is probably the best if anxiety or agitation is part of your depression, and Luvox® if you've been diagnosed with obsessive compulsive disorder (OCD). Newly available escitalopram (Lexapro®) possibly has less side effects than other SSRIs.

How does your doctor choose which one to use?

Because the SSRIs and tricyclics have a long track record and are relatively inexpensive, most health care practitioners continue to use them as first line agents for treating depression.

Match your symptoms profile to the drug's spectrum of effects. Make sure your practitioner explains to you what (s)he is giving, why, and what to expect.

It's probably best to maximize the dosage of whatever drug is used first before switching. Also, continue with the first drug for up to 12 weeks before you give up on it. Your goal is full (not partial) remission of symptoms and once remission has occurred, treatment should continue for at least 6-9 months. If you discontinue usage, make sure that you slowly taper off (over a month or more).

A mixed group of drugs called "new antidepressants" (some aren't so new) is gaining a substantial place in the medical armamentarium.

Venlafaxine (Effexor®; Effexor-XR®) is most commonly utilized as a second-line agent, especially with generalized anxiety disorder accompanying depression. It has no adverse effects on sleep and can actually be utilized for diminishing insomnia. It may have an adverse effect on sexuality. Nausea is the most commonly associated side effect, although treatment may be associated with increases in blood pressure. The extended release formulation is generally preferred.

Bupropion (Wellbutrin®; Wellbutrin-SR®) is a popular second-line agent, especially as it has no negative effect on sexuality. It is frequently combined with other antidepressants to minimize their adverse sexual effects. It is especially helpful in patients who have a degree of attention deficit hyperactivity disorder, ADHD. It can cause insomnia in some if taken later in the day. It is associated with an increased risk of seizures in high doses. Bupropion® is also marketed as an aid in smoking cessation under the name Zyban®. At least 30% of patients lose 5 lbs or more on Wellbutrin®. Unless insomnia becomes an issue, the sustained formulation is preferred.

Netazodone (Serzone®) has become a common choice for patients with anxiety symptoms because of its somnolent effects. It is associated with more drug-drug interactions than the SSRIs and other antidepressants and may cause some dry mouth and dizziness, as well as sedation.

Mirtazapine (Remeron®) appears to increase serotonin in the brain. Although it can cause somnolence in some patients, it has little effect on sexuality. Weight gain and dry mouth are an occasional problem.

As a footnote, I should mention gabepentin (Neurontin®). Originally developed and used as an anti-seizure medication, it has found a solid place as an adjunct to other antidepressants in the second-line therapy of depression. Starting with 100 mg at bedtime, doses are rapidly increased as needed, at times as high as 1000-1200 mg. It aids with sleep and has a relatively benign side effect profile. It can be especially helpful in bipolar disorder.

Other anti-seizure medications (including Depakote® and others) are now utilized by psychiatrists as adjuncts in the treatment of difficult-to-manage depression. They generally have a low side effect profile.

It is important to note, if you have been on an old-time class of antidepressant known as "MAO inhibitors" (Nardil® or Parnate®), you should not combine them with other antidepressants and must be totally off for at least 2 weeks prior to using any of the above-detailed drugs.

*All great truths begin as blasphemes.*
—Anna Janaska
*New Roads, new ruts*
—G.K. Chesterton

# CHAPTER EIGHTEEN

## THE FUTURE

The future isn't what it used to be. Here's what's new and juicy on the "midlife horizon" (besides old age!).

### Genetics

Many recent findings in the areas of genetic markers and genes point to a future where genotypes (one's genetic composition) and risk markers might help identify particular women who are candidates for specific hormonal therapies, and those individuals in which to avoid certain treatments.

Women's health practitioners have already felt the clinical impact of intelligent drug design, with the introduction of estrogen-enhancing SERMS (especially raloxifene or Evista®, and others to come) for prevention of osteoporosis.

Recently, a specific genotype was found more commonly in women experiencing adverse cardiovascular events when placed on hormonal supplementation. Also, a specific estrogen receptor ("estrogen receptor alpha") was isolated in lower concentrations in normal breast tissue of an Asian population at low risk for breast cancer.

Patients with a strong genetic risk for ovarian cancer seem to benefit from birth control pills for the prevention of the more virulent types of ovarian cancer. And of course we already know that women with certain gene mutations (known as BRCA mutations) may ultimately benefit from chemoprevention therapy with tamoxifen.

These and other findings will enable health care practitioners to identify populations of women who should, or should not, have certain therapies, and which women are most likely to benefit from a given treatment modality.

### Hormones

Much of our understanding of the true long-term effects of hormonal supplementation, compared with non-supplemented populations, await results of studies in progress and others not yet begun.

The recent termination of an arm of one of the larger of these studies, the Women's Health Initiative or "WHI," has taught us much, but more importantly has left many questions unanswered.

This study was done with Premarin®, also known as conjugated equine estrogens (derived from pregnant mare's urine, which, I guess, you'd call a "natural" product) combined with Provera®. Provera®, or medroxyprogesterone acetate, is a strong, cheap, synthesized progestin (a progesterone-like substance) which is known for its suppressive action on adverse estrogen effects within the uterus. It also has the most adverse effects on cholesterol profiles, thereby to some extent counteracting estrogen's research-proven long-term beneficial effects on the heart.

The WHI study was terminated because, after 5 years, there was a trend (although not statistically significant) toward a slightly increased risk of breast cancer in older women who used the specific combination of Premarin® and Provera® for over five years. This study also showed that "...estrogens had no beneficial effects on cardiovascular health in post-menopausal women and, in fact, may have an adverse effect..."

But look closer: this study was done on post-menopausal women mostly over 60-a group that might be expected to have a higher risk of cardiovascular disease. It did not include symptomatic peri-menopausal women, a group which may have greater long-term cardiovascular benefit from hormone replacement therapy. The study discovered an adverse <u>short term</u> effect of Premarin® and Provera® on this group of women. And with its termination after 5 years, the study was not able to determine long-term beneficial effects of estrogen (if any) on the study population (an effect which other, longer, studies have shown).

And what about estrogen alone? What about estrogen with bioidentical progesterone (i.e., Prometrium®) and other progestins (e.g. norethindrone acetate, or NET), both of which have been shown to have less of an adverse effect on blood fats than Provera®.

What about other estrogens-especially the bioidenticial estradiol? And is there a difference (beneficial or detrimental) with different delivery systems, e.g., transdermal?

So much is unknown. All that is known is that estrogens (especially when combined with the cardiac-unfriendly Provera®) have an <u>adverse</u> short-term cardiovascular effect in women with already-existing cardiovascular disease, but probably have a <u>beneficial</u> long-term effect in this population and in their less cardiac-challenged "sisters." Also, it appears that long-term (5 years or more?) estrogen supplementation increases, in sensitive individuals, and probably in a dose-dependent manner, the risk of breast cancer.

But what about sub-populations of women? What about the other estrogens; about progesterone and the other progestins? What about estradiol, what about transdermal delivery systems that bypass the liver on their first pass through the body?

We just don't know. New studies are being designed or in progress that will give some answers, but it will take awhile (read: 10 years or more) before there is any truly meaningful data.

The future may not be what it used to be.

Considerable progress has already been made in our understanding of the effects of estrogen on brain structure and function. This emerging knowledge has significant implications on the design of future studies to advance our understanding of estrogen's role in brain aging and the development of degenerative disorders. This knowledge will have significant implications for menopausal hormonal management.

New Delivery Systems

Much work is in progress and several new systems are in the FDA pipeline, for <u>delivery</u> of hormone replacement therapy.

A new flexible estrogen-releasing vaginal ring has just been approved by the FDA as of May 2003, and is described at the end of Chapter 6.

Look for new intravaginal and pelletized slow-release "under the skin" hormonal sources in the future.

A nasal spray for delivery of HRT is being tested. The more choices women have as to delivery systems, the greater compliance can be expected.

Early studies on the intranasal route demonstrate that it is safe, effective and acceptable to post-menopausal women. Both estradiol alone and estradiol with progesterone may be administered in this manner, as a once-daily spray. In a recent study[1] comparing the intranasal route with the patch, women reported more satisfaction with the spray for effectiveness, convenience, discretion, speed of administration, etc., in addition to a lowered discontinuation rate.

Although combinations of estrogen and a progestin are found in pill forms, with the exception of Combipatch® (which has limited dosage regimens), there are a paucity of transdermal patch options combining estrogen with progesterone or a progestin for HRT. Expect this to change in the future, with the availability of a patch combining estradiol or ethinyl estradiol with levonorgestrol, a progestin with a long track record found in several birth control pills and in the progestin intrauterine device (IUD), Mirena®.

---

[1]"Intranasal HRT", Wattannnakumtornkul, Pinto, and Williams, <u>Menopause: The Journal of the North American Menopause Society</u>, 2003, Vol. 10, pp 88-98

Estrasorb®, a topical emulsion of micronized bioidentical estradiol is presently being tested. If FDA approved, it would be the first non-patch topical estrogen replacement available outside of a compounding pharmacy.

Changes in Progesterone/Progestin Therapy

Progesterone or a progestin is usually added to the estrogen in HRT to protect the uterine lining (endometrium) from a higher incidence of cancer seen when long-term estrogen is administered alone.

This research, however, was conducted with higher doses of estrogen than the more minimal dosages presently available, and some of its methodology is suspect.

While the benefits of progesterone use in HRT are well recognized as far as endometrial protection is concerned, their cardiovascular risks and drawbacks are a concern.

Research is being conducted utilizing different progestins. Natural progesterone and some of its derivatives such as Nesterone® and others, and newly synthesized molecules such as drospirenone (the progestin found in the birth control pill Yasmin®) do not have masculine-producing side effects and have less of a deleterious effect on blood fats(lipids).

There is also a re-thinking taking place regarding whether progesterone or progestin supplementation of HRT is really necessary at all.

Recent studies have indicated that low dose estrogen replacement therapy (ERT) has been associated with a low risk of abnormal endometrial changes and a rate of endometrial (uterine) cancer not unlike that of "never-users."

Furthermore, most of the reports that relate ERT to an increased risk of uterine cancer show this to be predominantly low grade disease, casting doubt on the ability of ERT to cause high grade or more dangerous types of carcinoma.

The majority of the benefits offered by estrogen supplementation are related to quality of life and may, in some, lead to long-term use. Frequently, the systemic progestin (but not necessarily natural progesterone) effects lead to a potential reduction in the benefits of hormonal supplementation.

In the future, randomized trials of low-dose estrogen only vs. estrogen supplementation plus progestin will be carried out. Until this can be accomplished, less systemically adverse ways of progesterone administration would be to use natural progesterone, to use only 10-14 days of a progestin every 3 months, or to insert a progestin-impregnated IUD such as Mirena® (giving local uterine protection without adverse systemic effects).

New SERMS: Tibolone

SERMS (Selective Estrogen Receptor Modulators) may be the nearest thing available to the hormonal holy grail.

We've already discussed much on the only presently available SERM utilized for peri- and post-menopausal osteoporosis prevention and therapy. Although raloxifene has excellent effects in preventing bone loss, as well as generally beneficial effects on lipids and decreased rates of breast cancer, it does not improve sex drive and is not of help dealing with the disturbing symptoms of (peri-) menopause. (The ideal SERM would, like raloxifene, have beneficial effects on bone density and offer breast cancer protection while also alleviating peri-menopausal symptoms and conferring favorable effects on sex drive.

Does such an animal exist??

Much research has been done on tibolone, a synthetic steroid and SERM already used extensively throughout Europe and Asia for almost 2 decades under the trade name Livial®, for management of climacteric symptoms (trouble sleeping, mood swings or memory problems) with the proposed additional benefit of improving libido.

Tibolone alleviates post-menopausal vasomotor symptoms (hot flashes) without stimulating the endometrium. Hence, a progestin is not required and cyclical bleeding is not induced.

Tibolone has been shown to relieve vaginal discomfort and dryness and this may also contribute to the improvement in sexual desire seen with tibolone.

Tibolone also significantly lowers sex hormone binding globulin (SHBG) and increases circulating free testosterone, having androgen-like favorable affects on mood and libido.

Via its metabolic byproducts, tibolone has progestogenic, estrogenic and androgenic activities. It relieves hot flashes, improves urogenital atrophy (a loss of the tissue that lines the vagina or the bladder) and sexual wellbeing and protects bone. It does not stimulate the breast and has less breakthrough bleeding than ERT/HRT.

Although tibolone appears to have a beneficial effect on aortic compliance (stretchability), it does not appear to help the pliability of coronary arteries; however, some studies suggest that tibolone may have direct effects that offer protection against ischemia (diminished blood flow) in the heart. Some lipid parameters are favorably affected (lowering of triglycerides and lipoprotein-A); others are unfavorably affected, such as lowering of high density lipoproteins (HDLs).

Susan Davis, a major researcher in the area of hormonal therapies, recently published a review of all the published data on the effects of tibolone on sexual parameters, mood, and cognitive function in post-menopausal women.[1]

Tibolone increases beta endorphin levels in the blood, leading to improvements in mood. Tibolone's mildly androgenic effects may also lead to greater energy and mood improvement. Tibolone's effect on mood, however, may not be quite as good as that achieved with estrogens. Tibolone's greater improvement in libido and other aspects of female sexuality and enjoyment than conventional HRT is probably because of its combined estrogenic, androgenic, and SHBG-lowering effects.

The adverse effects of tibolone have not been totally addressed in placebo-controlled trials in this country. (Many of the trials compared tibolone with standard estrogen-progestin therapy and not with untreated women.)

Long-term usage in Europe and Asia has not uncovered any significant problems. Although, as discussed above, tibolone appears to meet, to a greater or lesser degree, all of the criteria for "the holy grail," many researchers feel that, until large placebo-controlled trials are conducted in this country, they cannot give it their official blessing, especially in areas of long-term effects in reducing fractures, diminishing breast cancer rates and coronary vascular disease.

Other SERMs are in the research pipeline, but none as far advanced (or with as much experience) as tibolone. Two of these compounds (levormeloxifene, idoxifene) have, in early phase 3 (human) testing been found to have problems in the area of increased urinary incontinence and other urinary problems, swelling of the uterine lining, uterine enlargement and abdominal pain, and further studies are necessary to see if these are causally related or just incidental.

Another SERM, "SCH57068" from Schering Plough, is in Phase 2 (animal) trials and appears to prevent bone loss, enhance bone mechanical strength, prevent elevation of cholesterol and LDL levels and block estrogen stimulation of the uterus in castrated female rats.

According to H.J. Kloosterboer, Ph.D.[2], project manager for HRT research for Organon, the manufacturer of tibolone (Livial), which has been in the FDA pipeline for years, tibolone was expected to be available in the USA during the spring of 2003. It has not yet gained FDA approval. Whether this is due to the uncertainties mentioned above, or because of

---

[1] "The Effects of Tibolone on Mood and Libido," Susan R. Davis, M.D., *Menopause: The Journal of the North American Menopause Society,* 2003, Vol. 9, pp 162-170.
[2] Personal Communication, October, 2001

intense lobbying from other pharmaceutical companies that certainly stand to lose a significant market share when tibolone becomes available, is speculative.

Testosterone

The big news in the area of androgen supplementation is the expected availability in the near future of commercially available testosterone supplements in female-friendly doses. (In following the availability, proper dosage and FDA approval of medications designed specifically for female use, one comes to the conclusion that, as seen in other areas of society, research on and availability of female-specific medication lags behind that for males.)

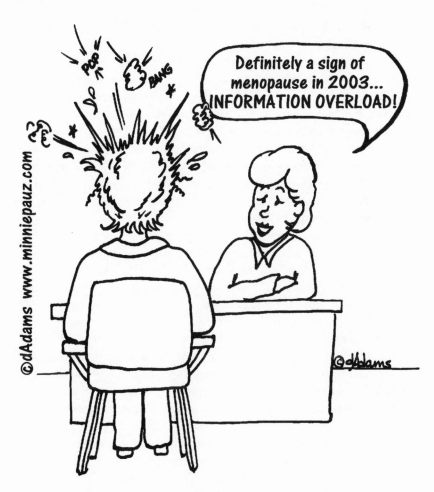

In addition to a metered testosterone spray being researched in Australia, at least two new drugs are in phase 2 or phase 3 FDA trials.

A testosterone patch, available in 3 dosages, should soon (translation: within the next year) be available from Proctor & Gamble. Look for it.

Androsorb, a topical emulsion of nanoparticles (super small particle size, designed for easy skin absorption) of testosterone in oil, produced by Novovax, Inc., is undergoing FDA trials. (The same idea, but using estradiol particles and known as "Estrasorb®" is also in the pipeline.)

## Bone Density News

Several "me too" drugs in the class of bisphosphonates (drugs like Actonel® and Fosamax®) and SERMs are being developed and will, I'm sure, be soon on the market. More choice, but more confusion.

Research is also being done evaluating the place for utilizing presently available medication such as a bisphosphonate (Fosamax®, Actonel®) with a SERM such as raloxifene (Evista®) or tibolone, utilized either sequentially (alternating one with the other) or in combination to see if this method of administration has more favorable effects on bone density than either method alone. Preliminary data suggests that this is so.

Some new drugs are being tested:

Another bisphosphonate, zoledronic acid, is in phase 3 studies. Zoledronic acid is administered intravenously every 3 or 6 months (a distinct advantage to daily or weekly oral dosing) and, in preliminary studies, appears to affect bone density in about the same degree as oral bisphosphonate therapy.

As discussed above, several SERMs are in phase 2 and phase 3 trials. Exemestane, in phase 2 trials, shows a potent effect in preventing bone loss, enhancing bone strength and preventing elevation of cholesterol and LDL levels in castrated female rats. Phase 3 trials are needed to support the safety of exemestane in post-menopausal women.

## Breast Cancer

Ductal lavage (a breast test for collecting cells from inside your milk ducts to see if there are any cells that are abnormal), although still little-used, has been on the medical scene for a couple of years. In this test, conducted on women with a high risk of breast cancer, a fine catheter is actually threaded into the milk ducts and cells are lavaged (or "rinsed out"). Unfortunately, only women who have open ducts (i.e., can express fluid with manual pressure) are candidates for this procedure.

The finding of abnormal cells on lavage indicates that something abnormal is going on, but provides no information particularly about where within the sample duct the abnormality is located, or even if a definable lesion is present.

This is where a new procedure, mammary ductoscopy, holds promise and may provide the missing link that renders ductal lavage clinically more relevant.

Ductoscopy is performed by threading a very slender endoscope (like a tiny telescope) into the duct and directly visualizing the duct lining to tell if a lesion, if present, is worrisome and warrants surgical excision.

As discussed in Chapter 10, the estrogen receptor is emerging as an important target for the treatment and prevention of breast cancer. Highly effective hormonal manipulations for breast cancer prevention and treatment are currently available (tamoxifen; probably raloxifen), but much more is being learned about these types of SERMs (called "aromatase inhibitors," aromatase being the enzyme responsible for estrogen synthesis in both normal breast tissue and breast tumors).

Depending on their chemical structures, these "aromatase inhibitors" are either steroidal (such as exemestane and formestane) or non-steroidal (such as letrozole, vorozole, and anastozole). These compounds' role in the treatment of advanced breast cancer is already well established.

Getting into some deep biochemistry here... The bottom line is that a lot of research is being done into compounds which manipulate hormones and their sometimes abnormal cellular growth-enhancing effects on breast tissue.

Genetic testing remains an important area of research in the prediction and prevention of breast cancer.

A new test, developed by Dutch researchers, utilizes a 1"x 3" computer chip to examine which of 25,000 genes were "turned on," or "expressed," in tumor samples from almost 300 women, all younger than 53. They discovered 70 genes that, when turned on or off in a certain pattern, predict whether the cancer will spread and kill the patient, thus delineating a higher risk group among women with breast cancer. The 10-year survival rate in the low risk group was 95%. The high risk patients were five times more likely to have their cancer spread.

This genetic test was much more accurate than the presently utilized methods in predicting recurrences of cancer, thus identifying women who would most benefit from intensive, invasive chemotherapy. The genetic test would put 61% of the women in the high risk category, compared with 90% under standard American methods, thus reducing the number of women getting chemotherapy by a third.

The estimated cost of this genetic test is roughly $1500. A round of chemotherapy would typically cost several thousand dollars or more.

The impressive thing about this type of work is the implication that many more of these types of things (advanced genetic diagnoses) are yet to come.

Most promising is a new methodology called "proteinomics" which, with computer assistance, allows researchers to analyze hundreds of specific proteins produced by cells to identify patterns or "fingerprints" distinctive to breast cancer. Looking at these proteins may help in much earlier diagnosis and may enable scientists to tell which proteins are likely to respond to various treatments. "Proteinomics" looks for proteins particular to the cancer or normal proteins at highly increased levels because of the disease. The idea is to identify a "protein fingerprint" of breast cancer for both diagnosis and disease-specific treatment.

## Lipid Lowering Agents

Marketing approval is anticipated soon for two new agents, rosuvastatin (Crestor®), a drug that like atorvastatin (Lipitor®), lies at the high end of the LDL-lowering potency spectrum, and ezetimbe (Zetia®). The latter is interesting because it affects cholesterol transport in the gut and because, in combination with taking a statin, results in a further 20% LDL level reduction, equivalent to a threefold boost in a patient's statin dose.

## Ovarian Cancer

Genetic researchers continue to work on identifying culprit genes in high-risk individuals, both for identifying candidates for increased surveillance as well as possible genetic manipulations.

The search continues for an inexpensive blood test to detect ovarian cancer. Most recently, a test which measures a hemoglobin (blood cell)-binding protein called haptoglobin-A has shown promise. Perhaps more promising is a serum (blood) test based on proteinomics, similar to that described above for breast cancer, but which is specific for ovarian cancer.

## Pelvic Floor

The big news here, of course, is that the less invasive mechanical slings of TVT (a vaginal "tape") and Stratasis (a urethral support) are showing excellent long-term results.

The newest promising thing on the horizon is the continued work on the pelvic floor from above, via laparoscopy, rather than from below through the vagina.

Traditionally, most all pelvic floor reconstruction for prolapse, cystocele, rectocele, enterocele and uterine or vaginal prolapse was approached via the vagina. Now, advanced laparoscopists and some urogynecologists are beginning to perform the same operations less invasively via the laparoscope, suspending and elevating from above rather than building a new floor below. Preliminary follow-up shows equal or better results with less trauma to the patient. Ask an advanced laparoscopist in your community, or check with the AAGL (American Association of Gynecologic Laparoscopists) (<http://www.aagl.org>).

## Fibroids

Less invasive surgical methods ("tying off" or occluding the uterine arteries laparoscopically or vaginally; "freezing" or cauterizing them by means of "Laparoscopic Forks," or "myolysis") and radiological methods ("uterine artery embolization") are available for those who absolutely do not want to lose their uterus.

Drugs are being investigated which non-surgically treat the excessive bleeding caused by symptomatic fibroids.

Asoprisnil (now in Phase III, or human, FDA trials), unlike Lupron®, the present "gold standard" medication for "shrinking fibroids," does not induce a hypoestrogenic state with resulting hot flashes and bone density loss.

A selective progesterone receptor modulator (SPRM), asoprisnil is thought to work by inhibiting blood flow at the endometrial level, thus significantly reducing the excessive bleeding associated with leiomyomas ("fibroids").


This is merely a taste of what's in the hopper and on the horizon and is, by no means, a complete list. Within the confines of time and available funds (think of what could be accomplished if we put a fraction of the money utilized to develop new weaponry into medical research), the search goes on.

*As long as you are trying to be something other than what you actually are, your mind merely wears itself out. But if you say, 'This is what I am; it is a fact that I am going to investigate, understand,' then you can go beyond.*

—Krishnamurti, in *The Penguin Krishnamurti Reader*

*Life is like playing a violin in public and learning the instrument as one goes on.*

—Samuel Butler

# CHAPTER NINETEEN

## THE FINAL CHAPTER
## Living Well with What You've Got

If I had to sum up midlife (...? life in general) in a phrase, it would be: "There is always a way."

I hope I've succeeded in presenting the facts and ideas to educate you to be able to work by yourself or with your health care practitioner to find that way.

Of course, that collaboration is easier and more fruitful if you have a savvy, non-biased practitioner who takes the time to work things out—your way.

But that's not always the case.

How can you find the right practitioner for you? How can you make your time together most productive?

1. Read and educate yourself before consulting with your health care practitioner. Not just one book, especially if it's by a "true believer" who touts "only one way" and denigrates the rest. See Chapter 20 for many good ideas.

2. Make your own list of questions before you go in. Better yet, write a short (but not over one page) narrative of your problems, your feelings, your concerns, your successes and failures, and what you want to accomplish and present it to your practitioner. If (s)he appears "antsy" and threatened by the list, find someone else.

3. Demand the time to work on this. You may need to do the discussing and arranging in 2 or 3 visits (not including follow-up checks) and you should not have to wait months for a working treatment plan.

4.   If the therapy is not working (and you've given it enough time), you may need to readjust or possibly see another practitioner. In fact, it may be very satisfying and cost-effective in the long run to pay the necessary money out of pocket to see a trained and certified menopause practitioner (medical doctor, M.D.; osteopathic doctor, D.O.; or a nurse practitioner, N.P.) to coordinate a therapeutic protocol or answer your questions, taking this information to your primary care physician for actualization. A few hundred dollars may save you months of anguish.

I often find it amazing that people will easily drop $100 on a dinner, $200 on clothes or a makeover, or $500-$1000 on a TV, but are loathe to spend a few hundred extra bucks on their health, comfort, and peace of mind. It's the mentality of "Well, my insurance is supposed to cover it." Well, if that insurance is an HMO, especially if that HMO is capitated (meaning that care providers are paid a flat rate regardless of services

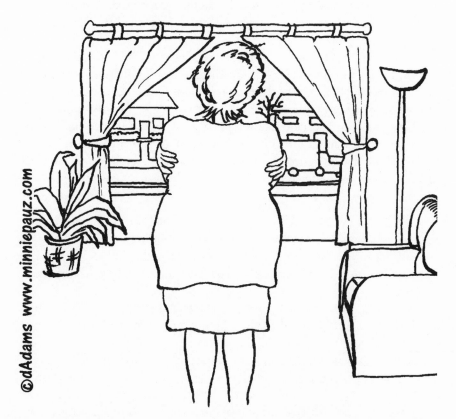

**Sometimes you just have to hug yourself!**

rendered) and you want something other than "Take two Premarin® and call me in the morning," forget about it.

In this area (as in so many others), you get what you pay for.

That said, where can you go to find a good practitioner?

Phone your local county medical society. Is there someone in your community (or close) who specializes in peri-menopausal medicine?

The North American Menopause Society (NAMS) has a web site (http://www.menopause.org) which lists all of its members (who, one would suspect, are at least interested in menopausal problems). Unfortunately, a number of these people are not clinical practitioners. Better is to check out those practitioners "highlighted," who are certified menopause practitioners or clinicians. If you live a long distance from the nearest competent practitioner, some will, after a visit in person, consult with you on-line or by telephone.

Additionally, visit the menopause/midlife sites on the Internet. There are many of these. Check your search engine (key words: "menopause," "midlife"). See which names appear on more than one list. These are the people to call.

Learn the "system savvy" diagnoses to suggest to your doctor to use to get the tests you need. These are the "insurance friendly" words to put in the "diagnosis" box on the lab/x-ray request form. It's a weird system. Although you may be at extremely high risk, e.g., for osteoporosis, or cardiovascular disease, you cannot put down "rule out osteoporosis" or "rule out abnormal lipids." You must write in an actual diagnosis. And it must be one that the entry-level coder who gets the billing slip can easily type in and is computer-friendly, to pay for the test in question. Here are a few examples:

> DEXA: "Over 65, not on HRT"; "Osteoporosis"; "Family history Osteoporosis"; "premature menopause"; "long-term use of high risk medications"; "follow up exam-osteoporosis"
> Lipids and Cardiac Testing: "hyperlipidemia"; "family history heart disease"
> Complicated Hormonal Testing: "menopausal symptoms"; "fatigue"
> "Second Level" Thyroid Studies: Immunological Tests: "fatigue"; "joint pain"; "hypothyroidism"
> Urinary Calcium Excretion Tests: "osteoporosis"; "hyperparathyroidism"
> Yearly Ultrasound for Ovarian Cancer Screening: "family history ovarian cancer"; "family history breast cancer and colon cancer"; "ovarian mass" (this diagnosis may be used for a yearly screen, as stool in the colon can always mimic an ovarian mass)

If you are at risk, you should have these and other screens. This is part of looking after your body and your health (along, of course, with a lifestyle plan that includes stress reduction, exercise, dietary awareness, calcium, smoking cessation, etc.).

Insurances do not pay for "rule-out" diagnoses (although, of course, that is what you are trying to accomplish). Sometimes you have to guide your health care practitioner "through the system" to get the care that you deserve!

Remember, this is about insurance. These companies are <u>not</u> in your corner. They are around for one reason only: to make money for themselves and their stockholders. You are merely the means by which they are able to do this. Remember also: the less care they provide, the less tests they authorize, the less medications they pay for, the more co-pays you are required to pay, the MORE MONEY THEY MAKE.

Unfortunately also, the present managed health care system (especially if you are in a capitated plan where the incentive is to <u>not</u> provide care) makes it difficult or impossible for many physicians to have the time and incentive to be an ombudsman for their patient, truly looking out for your best interests.

With very notable exceptions, <u>you are in this alone</u>. You must educate yourself and stand up and demand the care you deserve. (Through the ballot box also!!!)

There are lots of people out there ready to take your money in the area of peri-menopausal health care. Beware the false labels of "natural," "non-hormonal," etc.

Do you <u>really</u> know all that's in that supplement?? Each ingredient? At what dose? Is the advertised dose actually present? What it's supposed to do? How safe it is alone and combined with the other ingredients? Has anyone ever studied the long-term effects?

WHAT ARE YOU TAKING??

Aahhh...but it's "natural" (which is little more than an advertising buzz word).

It's amazing to me that people will not take a well-studied but perhaps synthetic medication which may cause a small number of known side effects, but will spend millions on products of which they know nothing (and about which little is known) just because they're "natural" or because a salesperson or web site says they are "<u>great</u>."

Also important: beware of the ol' "Bait and Switch" technique, which is alive and very well in the area of midlife health care. Beware the practitioner who comes on with "You don't need hormones; I only use natural products," and then prescribes "natural progesterone cream" or "bioidentical Bi-est or Tri-est cream," both of which have an excellent place in the peri-menopausal armamentarium, but <u>are in fact hormones</u>. One hundred percent. True, they are bioidentical (which I think is good). But, as you've read earlier, these are compounds, synthesized (no more, no less) from wild yam, soy, etc. to mimic, to be bioidentical with, the progesterone or the estrogen molecule found in "nature."

Midlife medicine has become a business and in business less-than-true advertising lures abound. I found a classic example recently in a quotation from a local nurse practitioner in a featured article on "Menopause" in a major high-end, glossy magazine named after the city (Sacramento) near where I practice. In the text of the article it states that "although [she] is licensed to prescribe traditional HRT medications, she does not." The text goes on to say that she "may prescribe estradiol patches, progesterone creams...and for [a specific patient] she prescribes a transdermal estradiol patch that slowly delivers a hormone made from plant sources..." Well, a hormone is a hormone. "Bait and switch."

Face it. You are (we are) aging. That is <u>not</u> a four-letter word! We can't stop that process (the claims of some web sites and "snake oil salesmen" notwithstanding).

The key is successful, healthy aging.

What are the components of healthy aging? Avoiding disease. Engagement with life. Maintaining a high level of cognitive and physical functioning.

Keep your brain functioning at its peak by taking on new and interesting challenges. Do crossword puzzles; learn to play a musical instrument; read more books; take an active role in community organizations. Go back to school and perhaps embark on a new career. Challenge your brain in new ways!

The more resilient you are, the more happily you will age. Do what you can to minimize stress. Now. Did you know that there is a positive relationship between holding anger in and the thickness of the arterial wall ("plaque") in many people? Anger/holding it in/stress = plaque. Did you know also that women with recurrent depressive symptoms have more plaque than their "mellower" sisters? The greater the history of recurrent depression, the greater the risk of coronary artery disease.

You don't have to <u>expect</u> to get depressed during "the pause" and then just "accept it." Gather the support of your friends (especially one or two good friends); engage the help of your health care practitioner.

The more you know about the process, the healthier you will be. Your goal? Making plans for the future. Having a sense of direction and purpose.

Continuing the process of learning. Gaining insight about life. Being secure and committed. Towards this end, a new book[1] is delightful. I highly recommend it.

With regard to midlife weight issues, it helps to understand some basic physiology. Because of the lowered amounts of growth hormone secreted from the adrenal glands (slowing your basal metabolic rate), women need to eat less and exercise more just to maintain a stable weight. A hassle, unfortunately, but "the way of life."

The midlife transition is your window of opportunity to be healthy as you age. Of course, paying attention to minimizing stress and promoting health is golden at any age, but it is in the early peri-menopausal years— THE MIDLIFE YEARS—that this window is open the widest.

Some final words on estrogen and progesterone.

A woman's most effective passage through midlife is to try and maintain a hormonal continuum (pre- and post-menopausally). The craziness, the depression, the stress comes from the disruption of this continuum. It is here that hormones, both synthetic and bioidentical non-hormonal compounds that have hormone-like effects, are most helpful, allowing you to maintain that continuum by giving you the tiller of your craft rather than having it bounce wildly out of control on the "peri-menopausal sea."

Understand also estrogen's effect on the breast and the cardiovascular system: High levels of estrogen over a prolonged period of time can disadvantage the breasts of a small number of women. Estrogen over even a short period of time can disadvantage a small number of women with pre-existing, significant plaque-containing coronary vascular disease.

The effects, however, of estrogens that are the most robust are in the inhibition of progression to increased plaque formation. While estrogen has a negative effect on established plaques, it has good effects in inhibiting atherogenesis (further plaque formation) over the long haul.

One statistic may be telling. The leading cause of death among women is heart disease (31%) compared to breast cancer, which accounts for 4% of death in women.

What about progesterone? The data is clear that progestins (especially medroxyprogesterone acetate or Provera®) have mildly adverse cardio-vascular effects. Certain breast tumors also have positive progesterone receptors.

---

[1]"Not Your Mother's Midlife. A Ten Step Guide to Fearless Aging," Nancy Alspaugh and Marilyn Kentz, Andrews McMeel, 2003

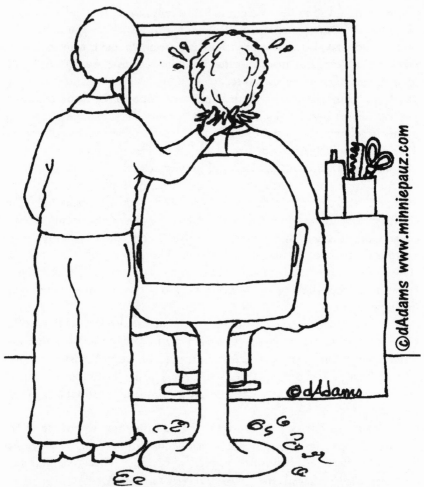

Well, Hans, I may not look 10 years younger or 10 lbs. lighter, but you definitely look $100 richer!

Micronized bioidentical progesterone, usually synthesized from wild Mexican yam root, whether by cream, lotion, capsule or troche, has a definite place in the tempering of the menopausal roller coaster. It remains to be seen if it truly does have all of the advantages and applications suggested by Dr. Lee[1] and others.

For better or for worse, most of us have a lot of life left to live (What's the alternative??). So: make it easy on yourself. You've got a lot of good knowledge and know about alternatives. Do what feels best for you at the moment. Don't feel stuck-there's plenty of time and room to "try on different shoes." Nothing is forever (...changing, changing...). You can switch lanes at will. There's always something new on the medical horizon.

It's up to you. You'll do it or you won't. Life will go on. In the end, there's only one person who controls the quality of your existence.

LIVE WELL WITH WHAT YOU'VE GOT! Hopefully this small book and the resources in the Appendix will help enable that.

EMPOWER YOURSELF. Be healthy. Feel good more often than not. Enjoy yourself. BE HAPPY!

---

[1] "What Your Doctor May Not Tell You About Perimenopause," John R. Lee, M.D., Jesse Hanley, M.D., and Virginia Hopkins, Warner Books, 1999

# CHAPTER TWENTY

## RESOURCES

This list could easily be twice as long as it is (I had to stop somewhere...). I truly hope the organizations, web sites, newsletters, books and references listed herein will educate and enable you to take the best path and make the best decisions about your health care.

Of course, feel free to browse the Net and your local book store for more ideas. A word of caution: beware single-outlook "only one way" sites and books, especially if they denigrate other approaches. *Caveat emptor!*

### USEFUL ORGANIZATIONS

About.com Women's Health Page:
http://womenshealth.miningco.com/nisub2.html

Alzheimers Association: 919 North Michigan Ave, Suite 1000, Chicago, IL 60611; (800) 272-3900; http://www.alz.org/

American Association of Retired Persons (AARP): 601 F St. NW, Washington DC 20049. http://www.aarp.org

American Cancer Society: (800) ACS-2345. http://www.cancer.org

American College of Obstetricians and Gynecologists (ACOG): 409 12th St. SW, Washington DC 20024-2188, (203) 638-5577 http://www.acog.org

American Diabetes Association: 1701 N. Beauregard St., Alexandria, VA 22311, (800) 342-2383. http://www.diabetes.org

American Heart Association: 7272 Greenville Ave., Dallas, TX 75231, (800) AHA-USA1. http://www.americanheart.org

American Menopause Foundation: 350 5th Ave. Suite 2822, New York, NY 10119, (212) 741-2398; http://www.americanmenopause.org

Female Patient: http://www.femalehealthlinks.com

Interstitial Cystitis Association, http://www.ichelp.com

National Menopause Foundation: 222 SW 36th Terrace, Gainesville, Florida, 32607, (800) MENO–ASK

National Osteoporosis Foundation, 1232 22nd St. NW, Washington, DC 20037-1292, (202) 223-2226; http://www.nof.org

National Sleep Foundation: 1522 K St. NW Suite 500, Washington DC 20005; (202) 347-3471; http://www.sleepfoundation.org

National Vulvodynia Association, P.O. Box 4491, Silver Spring, MD 20914, (301) 299-0775, http://www.nva.org.

North American Menopause Society (NAMS): P.O. Box 94527, Cleveland, OH 44104. Phone (800) 774-5432, http://www.menopause.org

Sexual Abuse
1) The Healing Woman Foundation, P.O. Box 28040, San Jose, CA 95259, (408) 246-1778.
2) VOICES in Action (Victims of Incest Can Emerge Survivors), P.O. Box 148309, Chicago, IL 60614, (800) 7-VOICE-8, http://www.voices-action.org.

Sexuality Information and Education Council of the U.S. (SIECUS), 130 W. 42nd St, Suite 350, New York, NY 10036. (212) 819-9770; http://www.siecus.org/ (A wonderful sex-information organization.)

Women's Health Interactive: P.O. Box 271276, Ft. Collins, CO 80527. http://www.nhlbi.nih.gov/whi/

## LABORATORIES OFFERING SALIVARY TESTS

Aeron Labs: 1933 Davis St., Ste 316, San Leandro, CA 94577. (800) 631-7900. http://www.aeron.com.

Diagnos-Techs, Inc: 6620 S 197th Pl. #J-104, Kent, WA 98032. (800) 87-TESTS. http://www.diagnostechs.com/

Great Smokies Diagnostic Lab, 63 Zillicon St., Ashville, Nevada City 28801-1074, (800) 522-4762, http://www.gsdl.com

National Biotech Lab: 3212 NE 125th St., Seattle, WA 98125. (800) 846-6285.

ZRT Lab, 1814 N.W. 169th Place, Ste. 3090, Beaverton, OR 97006, (503) 466-2445, http://www.salivatest.com

## PERI–MENOPAUSE, MENOPAUSE, AND HORMONAL SUPPLEMENTATION

### Web Sites

http://www.menopause.org
http://www.drnorthrup.com
http://www.miniepauz.com
http://www.nlm.nih.gov/medlineplus
http://seniorhealth.about.com

### Books

"The Change Before the Change (everything you need to know to stay healthy in the decade before menopause)," by Laura E. Corio, M.D., and Linda Kahn, Banam Books, 2000, $14.95.

An excellent comprehensive book. A great reference, it is well written and easy to read.

"Before the Change: Taking Charge of Your Menopause," by Ann Louise Gittleman, MS, CNS. Harper Collins, 1998, $14.95.

By a nutritionist and author of the best selling, "Beyond Pritikin." Explains peri–menopausal changes and offers a self-diagnosis quiz; the book includes a "changing diet" with tips and recipes that prevent and alleviate symptoms.

"Dr. Susan Love's Menopause and Hormone Book: Making Informed Choices," by Susan M. Love, M.D., Three Rivers Press, 2003, $15.95.

An excellent appraisal of the current post-NIH literature; scientific, but easy to understand.

"I'm Too Young to Grow Old: Health Care for Women After 40," by Judith Reichman, M.D., Time Books, 1997, $16.00.

A good, comprehensive book on peri–menopause and menopause; a bit dated.

"The Menopause Cookbook," by Hope Ricciotti, M.D., and Vincent Connelly, W.W. Norton & Co., 2000, $15.95.

Great recipes that your whole family will enjoy (don't read this book when you're hungry!)

"Menopause Guidebook," from North American Menopause Society, 2003, $10. Available from NAMS (800) 774-5342 or http://www.menopause.org or Amazon.com

A wonderful, succinct, unbiased, 60-page guidebook by NAMS, North America's preeminent non-profit scientific organization devoted to improving women's health through menopause and beyond.

"Menopause—The Complete Guide to Maintaining Health and Wellbeing and Managing Your Life," by Miriam Stoppard, M.D., D-K Publishers, 2001, $14.95.

An elegantly presented, very complete book. A "must read" for women who really want to know all about menopause.

"Menopause—The Silent Passage," by Gail Sheehy, Pocket Books (Simon and Schuster), 1998, $14.00.

An excellently written book, laid out differently than other books. It is as much as novella as a work of non-fiction.

"The Pause: Positive Approaches to Peri–menopausal and Menopause," by Lonnie Barbach, PhD. Plume Books (the Penguin Group), 2000, $13.95.

By the best-selling author with expertise in sexual behavior, this book emphasizes the diversity of menopause-related changes and options for dealing with them. It's called a "life-and-sanity-saving guide" and has wonderful vignettes.

"Peri–menopause: Preparing for the Change," by Nancy Lee Teaff, M.D., and Kim Writ, Prima Publications (Wiley), 1999, $14.95.

Provides useful recommendations for some of the common concerns of women regarding midlife changes; HRT discussion is a bit outdated.

"Screaming to be Heard: Hormonal Connections Women Suspect, and Doctors Still Ignore," by Elizabeth Lee Vliet, M.D., M. Evans and Company, Inc., First edition 1995, Second edition 2000, $29.95.

"The Wisdom of Menopause," by Christiane Northrup, M.D., Bantam Books, 2002, $18.95.

A well-written and complete guide, written from a personal space, providing a very thorough cover of peri–menopause and menopause.

## PMS

### Web Sites

http://www.pms.org.uk/ (National Assn for Premenstrual Syndrom - UK)
http://www.pms-journal.org/ (stories and poems by women about PMS)

## Books

"PMS and Peri–menopause Sourcebook: A Guide to the Emotional, Mental, and Physical Patterns of a Woman's Life," by Laurie Futterman, RN, PhD, and John Jones, PhD, Lowell House, 1997, $16.95.

A thorough discussion of PMS and the peri–menopause transition, written for women in their 30s and 40s.

"A PMS Self Help Book," by Susan Lark, M.D., Celestial Arts Press, 1999, $16.95.

Naturally-oriented book with good advice for PMS.

"SOS for PMS (whole food solutions for PMS)," by DeAngeles and Siple, Plume Books, 1999, $15.95.

A good cover on nutritional programs for PMS.

## MIDLIFE SEXUALITY

### Organizations, Web sites, catalogs, etc.

Betty Dodson's Workshops: P.O. Box 1933, Murray Hill Station, New York, NY 10156; http://www.bettydodson.com (excellent courses, videos, books, on self-stimulation and self-loving)

http://www.tantra.com

SIECUS, 130 W. 42nd St, Suite 350, New York, NY 10036. (212) 819-9770; http://www.siecus.org/ (A wonderful sex-information organization.)

Society for Human Sexuality, PMB1276, 1122 East Pike St., Seattle, WA 98122, http://www.sexuality.org.

### Excellent sources fo Catalogs, videos, books and sex toys

Eve's Garden (800) 848-3837; http://www.evesgarden.com
Good Vibrations (800) 289-8423; http://www.goodvibes.com
Xandria (800) 242-2828; http://www.xandria.com

### Books

"For Each Other: Sharing Sexual Intimacy," by Lonnie Barbach, PhD, Signet, 2001 (reissue), $7.99.

"For Women Only: A Revolutionary Guide to Overcoming Sexual Dysfunction and Reclaiming Your Sexual Life," by Jennifer Berman, M.D., Laura Berman, PhD and Elisabeth Bunmiller, Henry Holton Co., 2001, $15.00.

Written by sisters (one a urologist and one a psychotherapist), this book presents cutting-edge research and a comprehensive discussion of women's sexual issues; emphasizes the multiple causes of sexual problems. Excellent and informative.

"For Yourself: The Fulfillment of Female Sexuality," by Lonnie Barbach, PhD, Signet, 2000 (revised edition), $7.50.

"Getting the Sex You Want: A Woman's Guide to Becoming Proud, Passionate, and Pleased in Bed." by Sandra Leiblum, PhD and Judith Sachs, Crown Publishers, 2002, $23.95.

A discussion of women's sexual evolution and changes throughout the lifecycle, exploring sexual development and offering suggestions for changing and improving one's sexual awareness, behavior and satisfaction.

"Healing Love through the Tao: Cultivating Female Sexual Energy," by Mantak and Maneewan Chia, Healing Tao Publishers, 1991, $15.95.

From a centered, oriental perspective. As the title says...

"How to have Magnificent Sex: The Seven Dimensions of a Vital Sexual Connection," by Lana L. Holstein, M.D., Harmony Books, 2001, $21.00 (paperback $14.00, available December 2003).

An excellent resource with clear definitions, explanations, testimony, and gentle encouragement, it deals with feelings that can adversely affect sexual relations.

"I'm Not in the Mood": What Every Woman Should Know about Improving her Libido," by Judy Reichman, M.D., William Morrow, 1998, $12.00

"The Joy of Sex and More Joy of Sex" by Alex Comfort, Simon and Schuster, 1998, $40.00.

The classical wonderful-to-read and beautiful to look at "sexual cookbooks" exploring every pose and position imaginable.

"The Joy of Selfloving," by Betty Dodson, Crown Publishers, 1996 (reissue), $14.00.

A manual on self-pleasuring.

"The New Love and Sex after Sixty," by Robert N. Butler, M.D., and Myrna Lewis, PhD, Ballentine Books, 2002, $14.95

An informative and thorough book covering most every question 60-70-80 somethings may have regarding "...love and sex."

"Seasons of the Heart: Men and Women talk about Sex, Love and Romance after 60," by Zenith Henkin Gross, New World Library, (no date), $14.95

"Sex Smart: How Your Childhood Shaped Your Sexual Life and What to Do About It." by Aline Zolbrod, New Harbinger Publishers, 1998, $16.95.

"Turn Ons—Pleasing Yourself While You Please Your Lover," by Lonnie Barbach, PhD, Plume Books, 1998, $11.95.

** Also recommended are any of the erotic literature/short story collections edited by Lonnie Barbach, PhD.

## ALTERNATIVES ("COMPLEMENTARY AND ALTERNATIVE MEDICINE"; NUTRITION)

### Web sites

"Alternative Medicine Newsline": http://www.altmedicine.com

"Ask Dr. Weil": http://www.drweil.com

National Center for Complementary and Alternative Medicine: P.O. Box 7923, Gaithersberg, MD 20898, (888) 644-6226. info@nccam.nig.gov http://www.nccam.nih.gov

Natural Woman Institute, 8539 Sunset Blvd., Los Angeles, CA 90069, (888) 489-6626. http://www.naturalwoman.org. Founded by Christine Conrad, author of "A Woman's Guide to Natural Hormones."

### Compounding Pharmacies

College Pharmacy, 3505 Austin Bluffs Pkwy, Ste. 101, Colorado Springs, CO 80918 (800) 888-9358; e-mail: info@collegepharmacy.com.

International Association of Compounding Pharmacists (IACP), (800) 927-4227, http://www.iacprx.org/. IACP is a nonprofit organization that represents and serves over 1320 compounding pharmacists.

Kronos Compounding Pharmacy, 3675 South Rainbow, Las Vegas, NV 89103, (800) 723-7455, http://www.kronoscentre.com/compounding_pharmacy.aspx.

Rx Compound Centre, 1515 Hatcher Ln., Columbia, TN 38401 (931) 388-3999. Dr. Joel Hargrave's (The "father of Natural Progesterone") Pharmacy.

Women's International Pharmacy, 12012 N. 111th Avenue, Youngtown, AZ 85363, (623) 214.7700 - FAX: (623) 214.7708 or 2 Marsh Court, Madison, WI 53718, (608) 221.7800 - FAX: (608) 221.7819; http://www.womensinternational.com/

## Vitamins, Herbals, Bottanicals

PhytoPharmica ("Natural Medicines") (800) 533-3270, http://www.PhytoPharmica.com.

*There are <u>many</u> other reputable sources: ask your Health Food Store, naturopath or chiropractor.

## Books

"Professionals' Handbook of Complementary and Alternative Medications," by C.W. Fetro, Pharm.D. and Juan R. Avila, Pharm. D., Springhouse, 2001, approx. $20.

Written for healthcare professionals, it is an excellent resource on herbs, botanicals, and other alternative medications. It is a handbook, succinctly, yet thoroughly, describing all of these products. Recommended!

"Tyler's Honest Herbal," 4th Edition, by Stephen Foster and Varro E. Tyler, PhD, Haworth Herbal Press, 1999, $15.00.

An honest and investigative sourcebook for intelligent consumers desireous of straightfoward information on herbs and botanicals.

"Discover Your Menopause Type: The exciting new program that identifies the 12 unique menopause types and best choices for you," by Joseph Collins, N.D., Prima Publications, 2000, $16.95.

Individualizes therapy of menopause and menopausal symptoms, oriented towards alternatives methods. Not necessarily scientific.

"Estrogen the Natural Way: over 250 easy and delicious recipes for menopause," by Nina Shandler, Villard Books, 1998, $14.95.

Great recipes using foods with mild estrogen-like effects, such as soy and flax seeds.

"Menopause—The Natural Way," by Molly Siple, MS, RD and Deborah Gordon, M.D., John Wiley, 2001, $14.95

A nice, well-organized book on botanical, bioidentical and non-hormonal therapies of menopause. Highly recommended.

"Menopause without Medicine," by Linda Ojeda, PhD, Hunter House, 2000, $15.95.

A quite inclusive and excellent book offering natural alternatives but fairly presented and oriented toward health maintenance.

"Natural Hormone Balance for Women: LookYounger, Feel Stronger, and Life Life with Exhuberance," by Uzzi Reiss, M.D., with Martin Zucker, Pocket Books, 2001, $14.00.

An excellent reference on bioidentical hormones, especially compounded preparations.

"The New Integrative Approach: Menopause—How to Combine the Best of Traditional and Alternative Therapies," by Milton Hammerly, M.D., The Philip Lief Group, Inc., 2001, $7.95.

An excellent book covering the integration of traditional and alternative therapies.

"The Omega Plan: The life-saving nutritional program based on the diet of the island of Crete," by Artemus Simopoulous, M.D., Harper Collins, 1998, $11.20.

Summarizes research on healthy and unhealthy fats and the benefits of omega-3 fats found in fish, flax seeds, walnuts and green vegetables.

"The Soy Solution for Menopause: The Estrogen Alternative," by Machelle Seibel, M.D., Simon and Schuster, 2002, $14.00.Non-hormonal alternatives for peri–menopause and menopause, especially using soy.

"Super Nutrition for Menopause," by Ann Louise Gittleman, Publishers Group West, 1998, $12.95.

About "taking control of your life now and enjoying a new vitality with a diet/exercise program designed for menopausal women." A good reference for healthy nutrition.

"A Woman's Guide to Natural Hormones," by Christine Conrad, Peregree (Berkley—Penguin/Putnam) 2000, $13.95.

A wonderful natural hormone book; complete; answers all your questions.

"Women's Encyclopedia of Natural Medicine: Alternative Therapies and Integrative Medicine," by Tori Hudson, N.D., 1999, Keats Publishing, $24.95 (paperback).

Written by a leading naturopathic physician, this book presents a comprehensive overview of CAM.

## HEALTH, HEALTH ENHANCEMENT, EXERCISE AND WEIGHT

### Books

"About Your Cholesterol," American Heart Association, 2003, available free from the AHA (800) 242-8721.

A short (30-page) and simple guide to cholesterol, reflecting the AHA's latest recommendations.

"Kathy Smith's Moving through Menopause," by Kathy Smith, Warner Books, 2002, $15.95.

A concise, easy to read book by a leading fitness expert, especially for peri- and menopausal women.

"Outsmarting the Midlife Fat Cell: winning weight control strategies for women over 65 to stay fit through menopause," by Deborah, Mph Waterhouse, Hyperion, 1999, $12.95.

Fun-to-read weight control strategies for women over 35.

"Strong Women Stay Young," by Miriam E. Nelson, PhD, Bantam Books, 2000, $14.95

Excellent exercise reference.

"The Thirty Minute Fitness Solution: a 4-step plan for women of all ages," by Patricia Amand and JoAnn Manson, Harvard University Press, 2001, $22.95.

A practical easy-to-read book for both younger and menopausal aged women.

"Understanding and Controlling your High Blood Pressure," American Heart Association, 2001, free from the AHA (see above).

A 28-page booklet; simple and quick read regarding high blood pressure.

"Women, Weight and Hormones: A weight-loss plan for women over 35," by Elizabeth Lee Vliet, M.D., Evans and Co., 2001, $24.95.

An easy-to-follow, well-balanced book on the hormonal aspects of weight control.

## STRESS, MOOD, MEMORY, SLEEP ISSUES

### Web Sites

http://www.sleepfoundation.org/

## Books

"Healing Mind, Healthy Woman: Using the Mind-Body Connection to Manage Stress and Take Control of Your Life," by A.D. Domar and H. Dreher, Delta, 1997, $14.95.

A wide range of stress reduction approaches that help women manage the biochemical effects of stress. (Audiotapes also available).

"Improving Memory: Understanding and preventing age-related memory loss," by Harvard Health Publications, 2000, $16.00 (call (203) 975-8854, extension 106 to order)

"Improving Sleep: A Guide to getting a good night's rest," by Harvard Health Publications, 2002, $24.00 (call (617) 432-1485 to order)

"Menopause and the Mind. The Complete Guide to Coping with the Cognitive Effects of Peri–menopause and Menopause," by Claire Warga, PhD, Touchstone, Simon and Schuster, 1999, $14.00

Written by a neurophysiologist, this book identifies the "mind misconnect" problems that cause so many unsettling peri–menopausal and menopausal symptoms. A complete (if somewhat dense) text.

"Say Goodnight to Insomnia," by Gregg D. Jacobs, PhD, Henry Holt and Co., 1999, $14.00

Written by the developer of a behavioral medicine insomnia program, this book incorporates relaxation and other drug-free techniques to treat the thoughts and behaviors that cause sleep disorders.

"Self-Nurture: learning to care for yourself as effectively as you care for everyone else," by Alice D. Domar, PhD, Viking Press, 2000, $11.20.

From the director of Women's Health Programs at Harvard Medical School's Division of Behavioral Medicine, this book focuses on self-learning and offers meditation suggestions to assist the process of learning to care for yourself.

"Women and Sleep," National Sleep Foundation, 2001.

This 16 page booklet, published by the NSF is available free from the National Sleep Foundation (888) 673-7533.

"Women's Moods: What every woman must know about hormones, the brain and emotional health," by Deborah Sichel, M.D., and Jeanne Driscoll, MS, RN, CS, William Morrow and Co., 1999, $14.00.

An excellent resource on the connection between the female neuroendocrine system and mood, describing the evolution of hormonal changes throughout a woman's life.

## MIDLIFE: PHILOSOPHIC AND INSPIRATIONAL

### Web sites

http://www.fearless-aging.com
http://www.minniepauz.com

### Books

"Not Your Mother's Midlife: a 10-step guide to fearless aging," by Nancy Alspaugh and Marilyn Kentz, Andrews McNeel Publishing, 2003, $22.95.

A wonderful, clever, and eminently readable empowerment guide through and past menopause. Includes a meditation and visualization CD.

"If Not Now, When? Reclaiming ourselves at midlife," by Stephanie Marston, Warner Books, 2002, $13.95.

An up-beat book by a therapist with much of the author's personal commentary about her own midlife and those of women she has had in therapy.

"New Menopausal Years: the Wise Woman's Way," by Susun S. W, Ash Tree Publications, 2001, $12.95.

A beautifully written book interspersed with Native American wisdom. A glorification of aging, written from a very personal space. Some good advice is admixed with a prejudicial rejection of western ways and perhaps a blind embrace of things "herbal and natural."

"On Women Turning 50: Celebrating Midlife Discoveries," by Cathleen Rountree, Harper Collins, 1993.

A delightful timeless anthology of shared personal experience from well-known women describing their discoveries, life visions and feelings about growing older in prose and poems."

## POST MENOPAUSE AND AGING

### Web Sites

http://seniorhealth.about.com/
http://www.healthandage.com

### Books

"Aging Well: The Complete Guide to Physical and Emotional Health," by Jeanne Wei, PhD and Sue Levkoff, ScD, John Wiley and Sons, Inc., 2002, $17.95.

A complete, exhaustive and informative book on "aging well past 60."

"Ourselves, Growing Older (Women Aging with Knowledge and Power)," by Diana Laskin Siegal, Paula Brown Doress-Worters and Wendy Sanford, Touchstone (Simon and Schuster), 1994, $20.95.

A bit outdated, but a fine book on aging and later life, medical, social, political and economic aspects.

## BREAST HEALTH

### Web Site

Susan Love, M.D.: The Website for Women, http://www.susanlovemd.com

Y-Me National Breast Cancer Organization, http://www.y-me.org/

### Books

"Assess Your True Risk of Breast Cancer," by Patricia T. Kelly, PhD, Henry Holton Co., 2000, $15.00.

This book is a boon for women who are anxious or confused about their risk of breast cancer; it offers clear, well-documented information and guidance for decision-making.

"Dr. Susan Love's Breast Book," by Susan Love, M.D., and Karen Lindsay, Perseus Publications, 2002, $20.00

Written by a breast surgeon, this is widely considered to be the best consumer book addressing breast health and breast cancer.

## BONE DENSITY

### Organizations / Web Sites

Foundation for Osteoporosis Research (FORE), 300 27th Street, Suite 103, Oakland, CA 94612 (510) 832-2663, Toll free (888) 266-3015, Fax (510) 208-7174, http://www.fore.org

International Society of Clinical Densiometry (ISCD), 342 N. Main St., W. Hartford, CT 06117-2507 (860) 586-7563, Fax: (860) 586-7550, email: iscd@iscd.org, http://www.iscd.org/

National Osteoporosis Foundation, 1232 22nd St. NW, Washington, DC 20037-1292, (202) 223-2226; http://www.nof.org

NIH—Osteoporosis and Related Bone Disease National Resource Center, 1150 17th St. NW, Ste 500, Washington, DC 20036 (202) 223-2237 http://www.osteo.org

## Books

"Boning up on Osteoporosis: A Guide to Prevention and Treatment," by The National Osteoporosis Foundation, 2000. Available for $3 from the National Osteoporosis Foundation (877) 868-4520.

This excellent 70-page booklet is available from the nonprofit NOF, an organization devoted solely to improving osteoporosis prevention and treatment.

"Calciyum! Delicious Calcium-rich Dairy-free Vegetarian Recipes," by David and Rachelle Bronfman, Biomedia Books, 1998, $19.95.

...as the title says...

"The Osteoporosis Handbook: Every woman's guide to prevention and treatment," by Sydney Lou Bonnick, M.D., Taylor Publications, 2001, $14.95.

An excellent osteoporosis resource with well-researched information; very comprehensive and informative and a pleasure to read.

"Strong Women, Strong Bones: Everything you need to know to prevent, treat, and beat osteoporosis," by Miriam Nelson, PhD and Sarah Wernick, PhD, Putnam's Sons, 2000, $13.95.

A motivational and practical book by an exercise physiologist, it focuses on exercise, progressive weight training and the components of a "bone friendly" diet.

## PELVIC SUPPORT, INCONTINENCE, HYSTERECTOMY

### Web Sites and Organizations

Help for Incontinent People (HIP), P.O. Box 544, Union, S. Carolina 29379 (800) BLADDER

National Association of Continence, P.O. Box 8310, Spartonburg, SC 29305-8316, (800) 252-3337, http://www.nafc.org/

http://www.uterinefibroids.com

### Books

"The Incontinence Solution: Answers for Women of All Ages," by William H. Parker, M.D., Amy Rosenmen, M.D., and Rachel Parker, Simon and Schuster, 2002, $13.00.

Compact paperback full of practical information on the common and frustrating experience of urinary incontinence, genital organ prolapse, anal incontinence, interstitial cystitis, etc. Offers excellent informaton and solutions.

"Understanding Hysterectomy," American College of Obstetricians and Gynecologists, 1999.

This 12 page booklet offering basic information about hysterectomy is available free with a self-addressed stamped envelope from ACOG, 409 12th St. SW Washington, DC 20024, (800) 792-2264.

"The Urinary Incontinence Source Book," by Diane Kaschak Newman, RNC, CRNP, Mary K. Dzurinko and Ananias C. Diokno, Lowell House, 1999, $19.95.

Written by a urologic nurse, this book provides a comprehensive and detailed cover of urinary incontinence in women, men and children; includes self-help stragtegies.

## FATIGUE, FIBROMYALGIA, IBS, VULVODYNIA, ETC.

### Web Sites, Associations

1)  Fatigue, Fibromyalgia

http://www.fmnetnews.com
http://www.fibromyalgia.com
http://www.afsafund.org
http://www.drpodell.org/
http://guaidoc.com/

2)  Vulvodynia

National Vulvodynia Association, P.O. Box 4491, Silver Spring, MD 20914-4491 (301) 299-0775, http://www.nva.org.

TheVulvar Pain Foundation, P.O. Drawer 177, Graham, Nevada City 27252 (336) 226-0774, http://www.vulvarpainfoundation.org

3)  Interstitial cystitis

Interstitial Cystitis Assn. (800) HELP-ICA, http://www.ichelp.com

Good private site: http://www.ic-hope.com

### Books

"The Autoimmune Connection: Essential Information for Women on Diagnosis, Treatment, and Getting on with your Life," by Rita Baron-Faust, Jill Buyon, and Virginia Ladd, McGraw-Hill, 2002, $22.95.

An up-to-date, comprehensive book for women with autoimmune disease.

"Chronic Fatigue Self-Help Book," by Susan Lark, M.D., Celestial Arts, 1999, $16.95

"From Fatigue to Fantastic: A Proven Program to Regain Vibrant Health, Based on a New Scientific Study Showing Effective Treatment for Chronic Fatigue and Fibromyalgia," by Jacob Teitelbaum, M.D., Avery Penguin Putnum, 2001, $13.95

"The V Book: A Doctor's Guide to Complete Vulvovaginal Health," by Elizabeth Stewart, M.D., and Paula Spencer, Bantam, 2002, $13.95.

Complete and informative—everything you want or need to know about vulvovaginal problems and health.

## MISCELLANEOUS: HUMOR, WOMEN'S MEDICINE, MEMORY, GENERAL MENOPAUSE INFORMATION, LESBIAN HEALTH, MIDLIFE PREGNANCY, PREMATURE MENOPAUSE, ETC.

### Web Sites for Lesbian Health

http://www.lesbianhealth.net/
http://www.lesbian.org/lesbian-moms/health.html
http://www.glma.org/

### Books

"MenOpop," Fill'er Up Productions, Inc., http://www.menopop.com

The world's first menopause pop-up and activity book! A fun and loving way to introduce women to "The Change" and help them feel that they are not alone. Chosen by Dave Barry for his 2002 Holiday Gift Guide.

"A Gynecologist's Second Opinion: The Questions and Answers You Need to Take Charge of Your Health," by William H. Parker, M.D., with Rachel Parker, Ingrid Rodi, M.D., and Amy Rosenman, Plume, 2003, $15.

A quick but comprehensive review of a myriad of women's health issues, including midlife, with understandable drawings. Recommended.

"It's My Ovaries, Stupid," by Elizabeth Lee Vliet, M.D., Scribner, 2003, $28.00.

A kind of "Silent Spring" of women's health, this book covers dietary and food additives, lifestyle and environmental toxin factors affecting women's health in the areas of PCOS, premature ovarian failure, endometriosis, cystitis, allergies, mood disorders, fatigue, obesity, diabetes, hormone testing, etc.

"The Healthy Boomer: a No-Nonsense Midlife Health Guide for Women and Men," by Peggy Edwards, Miroslava Lhotsky, M.D., and Judy Turner, PhD, McClelland and Steward, 1999, $19.95.

An upbeat fact book with sensible advice and good anectdotes for both men and women at midlife.

"Hot Flashes, Warm Bottles," by Nancy London, MSW, Celestial Arts Press, 2001, $14.95.

Written by a therapist, it offers validation for "older" first time mothers at the same time approaching menopause.

"Menopaws: the Silent Meow," by Martha Sacks, Ten Speed Press, 1995, $10.95

A 64 page wimsical book using colored illustrations to present functional and fun hints for common menopause-related problems.

"Off the Rag: Lesbians Writing on Menopause," edited by Lee Lynch and Akia Woods, New Victoria Publishers, 1996, $12.95

These writings by lesbians on menopause give new insight about how some gay women feel about their reproductive function, sexuality, traditional medicine and menopause.

"Our Bodies Ourselves for the New Century: A book by and for women," by The Boston Women's Health Collective, Touchstone, 1998, $16.80.

A classic women's health primer and empowerment book with a strong feminist viewpoint to heighten your awareness.

"The Premature Menopause Book: When the Change of Life Comes Too Early," by Katherine Petras, Wholecare Publishers, 1999, $14.00

A personal account from a woman who has experienced early menopause. Chatty, informative and up to date.

"The Premature Menopause Guidebook," 2003, available from the North American Menopause Society (NAMS).

This 30 page resource is especially written for women experiencing early menopause from early ovarian failure or a medical intervention such as surgery, chemotherapy, or pelvic irradiation. Available for $10. Order directly from NAMS (800) 774-5432 or on line from http://www.menopause.org or Amazon.com.

"Sudden Menopause: Restoring Health and Emotional Wellbeing," by Debbie DeAngelo, RNC, BSN, Hunter House Publishers, 2001, $15.95.

A very good resource book on premature menopause, written by a nurse and health educator who had a early hysterectomy and oophorectomy at age 26 for ovarian cancer.

"Women's Body, Women's Wisdom," by Christiane Northrup, M.D., Bantam, 1998, $14.00

Big and somewhat daunting. Not truly a "midlife" book, but covers many health-related issues for women.

## NEWSLETTERS

**CAM:** Dr. Andrew Weil's Self-Healing: Creating Natural Health for your Body and Mind, Thorne Communications, Inc., 42 Pleasant St., Watertown, MA 02472 (800) 523-3296 or
http://www.drweilselfhealing.com. Cost: $18 per year, 12 newsletters.

**Nutrition:** Tufts University Health and Nutrition Letter: Your Guide to Living Healthier Longer. Available at $3 per copy from Tufts University, P.O. Box 420235, Palm Coast, FL 32142 (800) 274-7581,
http://www.healthletter.tufts.edu

**Herbs:** Herbalgram. American Botanical Council, P.O. Box 144345, Austin, TX 78714 (800) 373-7105, http://www.herbalgram.org. $50 annual membership; 4 issues.

### General

"A Friend Indeed." This "grandmother of all menopause newsletters" is available for $30 per year (6 issues) from A Friend Indeed, Main Floor, 419 Graham Ave., Pembina, ND 58271 (204) 989-8028,
http://www.afriendindeed.ca

"Harvard Women's Health Watch," $24 for 12 issues. P.O. Box 420068, Palm Coast, FL 22142 (800) 829-5921, http://www.med.harvard.edu

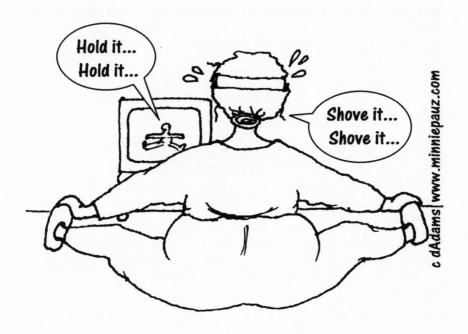

# BIBLIOGRAPHY

"Supernutrition for Menopause." Gittleman. Avery Publishing Group (1998).

A Comparison of Tibolone and Hormonal Replacement Therapy on Coronary Artery and Myocardial Function in Ovariectomized Atherosclerotic Monkeys. Williams, Hall, Anthony, Register, Reis and Clarkson. Menopause: The Journal of the North American Menopause Society (2002; 9: 41-46).

A Comprehensive Approach To the Menopause: So Far, One Size Should Fit All. Ewies. Obstetrical and Gynecological Survey (2001; 56: 642-49).

A Guest Editorial: Complementary and Alternative Medicine and Woman's Health—Time to Catch Up! Seibel (2003; 58: 149-151).

Add-Backs to Prevent Skeletal Fragility: Foresight or Folly? Editorial in Menopause: The Journal of the North American Menopause Society (2002; 9: 224-26).

Additive Effects of Raloxifene and Alendronate on Bone Density and Biochemical Markers of Bone Remodeling In Postmenopausal Women with Osteoporosis. Johnell, Scheele, Lu, Reginster, Need and Seeman. Journal of Clinical Endocrinology and Metabolism (2002; 87: 985-92).

Adverse Events Associated with the Selective Estrogen Receptor Modulator Levormeloxifene In An Aborted Phase III Osteoporosis Treatment Study. Goldstein and Nanavati. Presentation at 2001 meeting, North American Menopause Society.

Adverse Gynecologic Events Halt Research on Promising SERM. OB/GYN News (2003; page 22).

Alternatives to Conventional HRT: Phytoestrogens and Botanicals. Taylor. Contemporary OB/GYN (June 1999, pages 27-50).

Antidepressants. Jacobsen. Primary Care Update OB/GYNs (2002; pages 116-122).

Balancing Act. Slater. <u>Vogue</u> (June 2002 issue, 170-174).

Benefits of Soy Isoflavone Therapeutic Regimen on Menopausal Symptoms. Han, Soares, Haidar, Rodriguez deLima and Baracat. <u>Obstetrics and Gynecology</u> (2002; 99: 389-94).

Bone Density Screening for Osteoporosis. Committee opinion, <u>ACOG Committee on Gynecologic Practice #270</u> (March 2002).

Clinical Response as an Endpoint in Studies of Estrogen Replacement Therapy in Postmenopausal Women. Simon, Heuer, Schear and the Estrasorb Study Group. Poster Presentation at 2002 meeting, North American Menopause Society.

Comparison of Estrogen and Androgen Levels after Oral Estrogen Replacement Therapy. Slater, Zhang, Hodis, Mack, Boostanfar, Shoupe, Paulson and Stanczyk. <u>Journal of Reproductive Medicine</u> (2001; 46: 1052-56).

Controversy about Uterine Effects and Safety of SERMs: The Saga Continues. Goldstein. <u>Menopause: The Journal of the North American Menopause Society</u> (2002; 9: 381-384).

Current and Future Directions in Breast Cancer Care. Cauley. <u>The Female Patient</u> (supplement) (March 2002, page 13-18).

Delayed Childbearing and Its Impact on Population Rate Changes and Lower Birthweight, Multiple Births and Preterm Delivery. Taugh, Newburn-Cook, Johnston, Svenson, Rowes and Belik. <u>Pediatrics</u> (2002; 109: 399-403).

DHEA Can Boost Bone Density and Muscle Mass in Older Adults. <u>OB/GYN News</u> (April 1, 2002; page 26).

Diabetes and Menopause: A Special Population and Growing. Phillips. <u>OBG Management</u> (May 2002: 63-69).

Diet and Cardioprotection: Sorting Fact From Fiction. Krauss. <u>Menopause Management</u> (January/February 2002: 6-10).

Diet, Lifestyle and the Risk of Type 2 Diabetes Mellitus in Women. Hu, Manson, Stampfer, Colditz, Liu, Solomon, Willett. <u>New England Journal of Medicine</u> (2001; 345: 790-97).

Dietary Intake of Antioxidants and Risk of Alzheimer's Disease. Engelhart, Geerlings, Ruitenberg, Van Swieten, Hofman, Witteman et al. <u>JAMA</u> (2002; 287: 3223-9).

Discover Your Menopause Type: The exciting New Program That Identifies the 12 Unique Menopause Types and the Best Choices For you. Collins. Prima Publications (2002).

Drug Update: Lipid Modification for Secondary Prevention of Coronary Events. Clinical Rounds <u>OB/GYN News</u> (November 1, 2002; page 33).

Drug Update: New Antidepressants-beyond SSRIs. Article in <u>OB/GYN News</u> (March 1, 2002, page 24).

Ductoscopy, Lavage Combo Promising. Article in <u>OB/GYN News</u> (February 15, 2001).

Effect of Estrogen Replacement plus Low-Dose Alendronate Treatment on Bone Density in Surgically Postmenopausal Woman with Osteoporosis. Palomba, Orio, Colao, diCarlo, Sena, Lombardi, Zullo and Mastrantonio. <u>Journal of Clinical Endocrinology and Metabolism</u> (2002; 87: 1502-08).

Effect of Estrogen Replacement Therapy (ERT) On Daily Stress and Memory in Postmenopausal Women. Kraemer, Hollander, George, Kraemer, Javed, Ogden and Castracane. Paper presented at the 2001 annual meeting of the North American Menopause Society.

Effect of Exercise on Total and Intra-Abdominal Body Fat in Postmenopausal Women: A Randomized Controlled Trial. Irwin, Ysui, Ulrich, Bowen, Rodulph, Schwartz, et al. <u>JAMA</u> (2003; 289: 323-30).

Efficacy and Tolerability of a New Intravaginal Ring Delivering Estradiol Acetate Versus Placebo in Treatment of Vasomotor and Vulvovaginal Symptoms. Spiroff and Archer. Presentation at 2001 meeting, North American Menopause Society.

Estrogen Replacement Therapy For Menopausal Women With A History of Breast Carcinoma: Results of a Five-Year Prospective Study. Vassilopoulou-Sellin, Cohen, Hortobagyi, Klein, McNeese, Singletary, et al <u>Cancer</u> (2002; 95: 1817-26).

Estrogens Initiate and Promote the Growth of Breast Cancer. Goss. Paper presented at the 12th annual meeting of the North American Menopause Society (2001).

Fatigue and Pain You Can't Explain: Relief From Fibromyalgia. Podell. Article in <u>Bottom Line Personal</u> (April 15, 2003, pages 11-12).

FDA Approves Novel Osteoporosis Treatment: In OB/GYN News, (January 1, 2003: 4).

Focus on Primary Care: Thyroid Function and Dysfunction in Women. Aldersberg and Burrow. Obstetrical and Gynecological Survey (supplement) (2002; 57: S1-S6).

For Women Only: A Revolutionary Guide to Overcoming Sexual Dysfunction and Reclaiming Your Sexual Life. Berman, Berman and Bunmiller. Henry Holt Company (2001).

Gabapentin's Effect of Hot Flashes in Postmenopausal Women: A randomized controlled trial. Guttuso, Kurlan, McDermott, Kieburtz. Obstetrics and Gynecology (2003; 101: 337-45).

Genetics and Menopause: New developments to improve clinical outcomes. Shulman. The Female Patient (supplement) (December 2001, pages 3-6).

Ginkgo for Memory Enhancement. A Randomized Controlled Trial. Solomon, Adams, Silver, Zimmer and DeVeaux. JAMA (2002; 288: 835-40).

Gynecologic Care of the Cancer Patient. Castiel and Hoskins. OBG Management (January 2002, 37-49).

Healing Love through the Tao: Cultivating Female Sexual Energy. Chia and Chia (2001).

Healthy Bones 2002. Cosman, Stuenkel and Silverman. Seminar held at 2002 meeting, North American Menopause Society.

Herbal Management of Menopausal Symptoms. OB/GYN News (December 2001, page 18).

High Fish Consumption Key Road to Heart Health. OB/GYN News (March 1, 2002, page 26).

Homocysteine and Vascular Disease. Rubenstein. Lecture given at "Annual Update in Medicine," Stanford University School of Medicine (June 4, 2002).

Hormonal Manipulations and Breast Cancer. Benshushan and Brzezinski. Obstetrical and Gynecological Survey (2002; 57: 314-323).

Hormone Replacement In Breast Cancer: What Are the Connections? Speroff. The Female Patient (supplement) (December 2001: pages 6-12).

Hormone Replacement Therapy after a Diagnosis of Breast Cancer In Relation To Recurrence and Mortality. O'Meara, Rossing, Daling, Elmore, Barlow and Weiss. Journal of National Cancer Institute (2001; 93: 754-62).

Hormone Replacement Therapy and Incidence of Alzheimer's Disease In Older Woman: The Cache County Study. Zandi, Carlson, Plassman, Welsh-Bohmer, Mayer, Steffens, et al for the Cache County Memory Study investigators, JAMA (2002; 288: 2123-9).

Hormone Replacement Therapy: Trends in Formulations and Dosages. Portman. The Female Patient (supplement) (December 2001, pages 25-28).

Hormones and the Health of Women: Past, Present and Future (Keynote address at annual meeting of North American Menopause Society 2002). Menopause: The Journal of the North American Society (2002; 9: 23-31).

Hot Flash Trends and Mechanisms. Freedman. Editorial in Menopause: The Journal of the North American Menopause Society (2002: 9: 151-52).

HRT and Cognitive Function: What Are We To Believe? Birge. Editorial in Menopause: The Journal of the North American Society (2002; 9: 221-22).

HRT and Heart Disease: Making Sense of the Data. Villablanca. Lecture given at the Northern California OB/GYN Society (June 19, 2002).

HRT, dose and BMI. Utian. Menopause Management (supplement) (March 2002, pages 15-16).

Improving Your Skills in Managing Patients with Urinary Incontinence. Rosenman, Sweeting and Cornella. Postgraduate course at 2001 meeting of the American Association of Gynecologic Laparoscopists.

Indicators of Lifetime Estrogen Exposure: Effective Breast Cancer Incidence and Interaction with Raloxifene Therapy in the Multiple Outcomes of Raloxifene Evaluation Study Participants. Lippman, Kreuger, Eckert, Sashegyi, Walls, Jamal, Cauley and Cummings. Journal of Clinical Oncology (2001; 19: 3111-16).

Intranasal Hormone Replacement Therapy. Wattanakumtornkul, Pinto and Williams. Menopause: The Journal of North American Menopause Society (2003; 10: 88-96).

Intravaginal Ring Delivering Estradiol Acetate: Effect on Vulvovaginal Signs and Symptoms. Archer and Ballaga. Presentation at 2001 North American Menopause Society Meetings.

Intravenous Zoledronic Acid in Postmenopausal Women with Low Bone Mineral Density. Reid, Brown, Burckhardt, Horowitz, Richardson, Trechsel, Widmar, Devogelaer, Kaufman, Jaeger, Body and Meunier. New England Journal of Medicine (2003; 346: 653-61).

Long-Term Effects of Tibolone on Postmenopausal Monkeys: Evaluations of Multiple Tissues. Clarkson, Anthony, Cline, Lees and Ederveen. Presentation at 2001 meeting, North American Menopause Society.

Mammographic Changes in Women Undergoing Different HRT Regimens. Maamari and Schrieber. Paper presented at the 2001 annual meeting of the North American Menopause Society.

Managing Hot Flashes: Findings on Alternatives to Traditional Hormonal Therapy. Barton, Loprinzi and Ko. Menopause Management (May/June 2002 15-19).

Managing PMDD with SSRIs. Parker, Brown and Ling. OBG Management (March 2000, pages 67-71).

Menopause After Breast Cancer: How Women Cope. Knobf. Menopause Management (March/April 2002: page 8-12).

Metabolic Effects of Low-Dose ERT/HRT. Carr. Menopause Management (supplement) (March 2002, pages 13-14).

Micellar Nanoparticles: A New Topical Emulsion for Systemic Delivery of Estradiol and Testosterone. Heuer and Wright. Poster presentation at 2002 meeting, North American Menopause Society.

More Antioxidants, Less Fat May Curb Alzheimer's. OB/GYN News (November 1, 2002; page 32).

Multiple news letters from years 2001-2003 from NYA: The National Vulvodynia Association.

NAMS Physician Statement on Osteoporosis in Menopause: The Journal of the North American Menopause Society (2002; 9: 83-98).

New Anabolic Agent May Revamp Osteoporosis Therapy. OB/GYN News (May 1, 2002, page 20).

New Estrogen Guidelines: Two Experts Give Opposing Views. Love and Notelovitz. OBG Management (March 2003; 47-59).

New Intravaginal Ring Delivery of Estradiol Acetate Versus Placebo: Patient Acceptance and Effect on Climacteric Symptoms. Ballagh and Archer. Presentation at 2001 Meeting, North American Menopause Society.

New Options in Osteoporosis Therapy: Combination and Sequential Treatment. Barbieri. OBG Management (March 2003; 60-65).

New Perspectives on the Relationship of Hormone Changes to Affective Disorders in the Perimenopause. Vliet & Hutchseon. NAACOG's Clinical Issues (1991; 2: 453-58).

New Statement Defines Androgen Insufficiency. Article in OB/GYN News (July 1, 2002, page 18).

Not Your Mother's Midlife: The Ten-Step Guide To Fearless Aging. Alspaugh and Kentz. Andrews McMeel Publishers (2003).

NSAID, Aspirin Use Tied to Lower Incidence of Alzheimer's. OB/GYN News (December 15, 2002; page 34).

Obesity in Adulthood and Its Consequences For Life Expectancy: A Life-Table Analysis. Peeters, Barendregt, Willekens, Mackenbach, AlMamun, Bonneux, et al for the Netherlands Epidemiology and Demography Compression of Morbidity Research Group. Annals of Internal Medicine (2003: 128; 24-32).

Osteoporosis Drugs "Vastly Underused." OB/GYN News (December 1, 2002, page 18).

Osteoporosis: Fractures and Key Risk Factors. Dore. The Female Patient (supplement) (March 2002: 5-12).

Osteoporosis: Quality of Life and Diversity Issues. Barrett-Connor, Greendaale and McClung. Seminar held at 2002 meeting, North American Menopause Society.

Parathyroid Hormone for Osteoporosis Treatment: An Update. Bilezikian. Menopause Management (January/February 2002, pages 22-25).

Paternal Age and Risk of Schitzofrenia in Adult Offspring. Brown, Schaefer, Wyatt, Begg, Goetz, Bresnahan, Harkavy-Friedman, Gorman, Malaspina and Susser. The American Journal of Psychiatry (2002; 159: 1528-33).

Patient Preference and Compliance with Estrasorb, and Estradiol Topical Emulsion, In the Treatment of Symptomatic Postmenopausal Women. Heuer, Simon and Wright. Poster presentation at 2002 meeting, North American Menopause Society.

Pelvic-Support Defects: A Guide to Anatomy and Physiology. Julian. OBG Management (November 2002, pages 71-81).

Phase I Study of Topical Testosterone in Estradiol- and Testosterone-Deficient Postmenopausal Women. Heuer, Brisker, Muenz and Boxenbaum. Poster presentation at 2002 meeting, North American Menopause Society.

Postmenopausal Uterine Bleeding Profiles with Two Forms of Continuous Combined Hormone Replacement Therapy. Johnson, Davidson, Archer and Bachman. Menopause: The Journal of the North American Menopause Society (2002; 9: 16-22).

Premenstrual Syndrome and Premenstrual Dysphonic Disorder. Cronje and Studd. Primary Care Clinics In-Office Practice (2002; 29: 1-12).

Premenstrual Syndrome. ACOG Practice Bulletin #15 (April 2002).

Premenstrual Syndrome: Breaking Through the PMS Cloud. Krames Communications, San Bruno, California (1988).

Present Status of the Swan Study. Matthews. Presentation at 2002 meeting, North American Menopause Society.

Preservation of Bone Density in Postmenopausal Women. Abelson. The Female Patient (supplement) (December 2001: 20-24).

Prevalence of the Metabolic Syndrome Among US Adults: Findings From the Third National Health and Nutrition Examination Study. Ford, Giles and Dietz. JAMA (2002; 287: 256-59).

Professional's Handbook of Complimentary and Alternative Medicines. Fetrow and Avila. Springhouse (2001).

Progestagen Supplementation of ERT Really Necessary? Naftolin. Editorial in Menopause: The Journal of the North American Menopause Society (2002; 9: 1-2).

Progesterone Skin Cream and Measurements of Absorption. Gambrell. Editorial in Menopause: The Journal of the North American Menopause Society (2003; 10: 1-3).

Progestins in Hormonal Replacement Therapy: New Molecules, Risks and Benefits. Sitruk-Ware. Menopause: The Journal of the North American Menopause Society (2002; 9: 6-14).

Protein Could Be Marker Of Early Ovarian Cancer. Article in OB/GYN News (2003; page 12).

Reconstructive Surgery for Pelvic Floor Disorders. McKinney, Bent and Miklos. Postgraduate course at 2001 meeting of American Association of Gynecologic Laparoscopists.

Rise of TVT Shifts Focus from Laparoscopic to Vaginal Surgery. OB/GYN News (February 15, 2003, page 11).

Safety and Efficacy of a Continuous Once-A-Week 17 B-Estradiol/-Levonorgestrel Transdermal System and Its Effects on Vasomotor Symptoms and Endometrial Safety in Postmenopausal Women: The Results of Two Multicenter, Double-Blind, Randomized, Controlled Trials. Shulman, Yankov and Uhl. Menopause: The Journal of the North American Menopause Society (2002; 9: 195-206).

Safety and Side Effects of Low-Dose ERT/HRT. Archer. Menopause Management (supplement) (March 2002; 11-12).

Selective Estrogen Receptor Modulators. ACOG Practice Bulletin (Clinical Management Guidelines for Obstetrician/Gynecologist) #39, (October, 2002).

Sexual Counseling Made Simple. Smith. Resident and Staff Physician (1989; 35: 85-88).

Sexuality After Breast Cancer. Graziottin. Menopausal Medicine (2001; 9: 1-4).

Short-Term Use of Estradiol as an Antidepressant Strategy In Peri- and Postmenopausal Women. Cohen, Soares, Poitras, Schifren and Alexander. Paper presented at the 2001 annual meeting of the North American Menopause Society.

Sildenafil and Effective Treatment for Arousal Disorders in Premenopausal Women? Comment by Levy, OBG Management (April 2002, page 12).

Sleep Difficulty in Women at Midlife: A Community Survey of Sleep and the Menopausal Transition. Kravitz, Ganz, Bromberger, Powell, Sutton-Tyrrell and Meyer. Menopause: The Journal of the North American Menopause Society (2003; 10: 19-28).

Soy May Be Harmful in Women With Ischemia. OB/GYN News (May 15, 2002, page 14).

Sustained-Release Sodium Flouride in the Treatment of the Elderly with Established Osteoporosis. Rubin, Pak, Adams-Huet, et al. Archives of Internal Medicine (2001; 161: 2325-33).

Tension-Free Vaginal Tape: A Quality-Of-Life Assessment. Vassallo, Kleeman, Segal, Walsh, Karram. Obstetrics and Gynecology (2002; 100: 518-24).

Testosterone Treatment: Psychological and Physical Effects in Postmenopausal Women. Davis. Menopausal Medicine (2001; 9: 1-6).

The Effect of Behavioral Therapy on Urinary Incontinence: A Randomized Controlled Trial. Subak, Quesenberry, Posner, Cattolica, Soghikian. Obstetrics and Gynecology (2002: 172-78).

The Effectiveness of the Gail Model In Estimating Risk For Development of Breast Cancer in Women Under 40 Years of Age. McKarem, Roche and Hughes. Breast Journal (2001; 7 [1]: 34-39).

The Effects of Long-Term Tibolone On Aortic Compliance. Robinson, Millasseau, Chowienczyk and Rymar. Poster presentation at 2001 meeting of North American Menopause Society.

The Effects of Ten Years Tibolone Therapy on Endometrial Thickness. Bruce, Robinson and Rymar. Poster presentation at 2001 meeting, North American Menopause Society.

The Effects of Tibolone on Mammographic Density Over Ten Years. Bruce, Robinson, McWilliams, Fentiman and Rymar. Poster presentation at 2001 meeting, North American Menopause Society.

The Effects of Tibolone on Mood and Libido. Davis. Menopause: The Journal of the North American Menopause Society (2002; 9: 162-170).

The Experience of Menopause After Breast Cancer Therapy. Knobf. Presentation at 2001 meeting, North American Menopause Society.

The Incontinence Solution: Answers for Women of All Ages. Parker, Rosenman and Parker. Simon and Schuster (2003).

The Menopause Guidebook. The North American Menopause Society (2003).

The Physician's Desk Reference (PDR) 2003 Edition.

The Role of Androgen Therapy in Postmenopausal Women. Davis, Labrie, Shifran and Gass. Seminar at 2001 meeting, North American Menopause Society.

The Role of Androgen Therapy in Postmenopausal Women. Seminar. Labrie, Davis and Shifran. Seminar at 2002 meeting, North American Menopause Society.

The Role of HRT and SERMs: Evidence-Based Medicine. Nolan. The Female Patient (supplement) (March 2002; pages 3-4).

The Role of the OB/GYN in Evaluating and Managing Urinary Incontinence. Karram, Culligan and Fleischman. OBG Management (supplement) (April 2002).

The Selective Estrogen Receptor Modulator SCH57068 Prevents Bone Loss, Reduces Serum Cholesterol and Blocks Estrogen-Induced Uterine Hypertrophy in Ovariectomized Rats. Goss, Cheung, Pachter, Hu and Qi. Poster presentation at 2002 meeting, North American Menopause Society.

The Steroidal Aromatase Inhibitor Exemestane Prevents Bone Loss and Reduces Serum Cholesterol in Ovariectomized Rats. Goss, Grynpas, Lowery, Qi and Hu. Poster presentation at 2002 meeting, North American Menopause Society.

Tibolone For Postmenopausal Women: Systematic Review of Randomized Trials. Modelska and Cummings. The Journal of Clinical Endocrinology and Metabolism (2002; 87: 16-23).

Tibolone: Expanding Therapeutic Options. O'Connor, Kloosterboer, Gallagher and Thorneycroft. Symposium at 2001 meeting, North American Menopause Society.

Transdermal 1% Testosterone Cream Improves Mood, Wellbeing and Libido in Premenopausal Women. Goldstat, Tran, Briganti and Davis. Presentation at 2002 meeting, North American Menopause Society.

Transdermal Estradiol Reduces Plasma Myeloperoxidase Levels Without Affecting the LDL Resistance to Oxidation or the LDL Particle Size. Hermenegildo, Garcia-Martinez, Valldecabres, Tarin and Cano. Menopause: The Journal of the North American Menopause Society (2002; 9: 102-107).

Transdermal Progesterone and Its Effects on Vasomotor Symptoms, Blood Lipid Levels, Bone Metabolic Markers, Moods and Quality of Life for Postmenopausal Women. Wren, Champion, Manga and Eden. Menopause: Journal of North American Menopause Society (2003; 10: 13-18).

Treating Hot Flashes without Hormone Replacement Therapy. Seibel. OBG Management (May 2002, pages 70-81).

Treatment of Urogenital Atrophy with Low-Dose Estradiol: Preliminary results. Santen, Pinkerton, Connoway, Ropka, Wisniewski, Demers and Klein. Menopause: The Journal of the North American Menopause Society (2002; 9: 179-87).

Treatment with Percutaneous-Testosterone Gel in Women with Sexual Arousal Disorder-Effects on Quality of Life. Nathorst-B__s, Jarkander-Rolff, Carlstr_m and von Schoultz. Poster presentation at 2002 meeting, North American Menopause Society.

Trough Serum Levels of Estradiol, Estrone and FSH Following Topical Application of Estrasorb. Heuer, Utian, Schear, Wright and the Estrasorb Study Group. Poster presentation at 2002 meeting of North American Menopause Society.

Ultrasonographic Endometrial Thickness for Diagnosing Endometrial Pathology in Woman with Postmenopausal Bleeding; A Meta-Analysis. Gupta, Chien, Voit, Clark and Khan. ACTA OBSTET Gynecology Scand (2002; 81: 799-816).

Urinary Incontinence. What You Should Know About Urinary Incontinence. Patient Guide in OBG Management (December 2002, page 81-82).

Use of Botanicals for Management of Menopausal Symptoms. ACOG Practice Bulletin #28 (June 2001).

Wake Up Refreshed: How to Get To Sleep and Stay Asleep. Doghramji. Article in September 1, 2002 issue of Bottom Line Personal.

Weighing HRT Use after Breast Cancer. Creasman. OBG Management (June 2002; 16-32).

What is the Partner's Impact on Sexuality and Health Behavior in Women Around Menopause? Bitzer, Alder, DeGeyter and Holzgereve. Poster presentation at 2002 meeting, North American Menopause Society.

# INDEX